AN INTRODUCTION
TO EMS RESEARCH

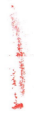

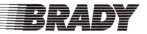

AN INTRODUCTION TO EMS RESEARCH

Lawrence H. Brown, EMT-P
Clinical Assistant Professor
Director of Research
Department of Emergency Medicine
SUNY Upstate Medical University
Syracuse, New York

Elizabeth A. Criss, RN, CEN, MEd
Base Hospital Manager/Clinical Educator
University Medical Center
Senior Research Associate
University of Arizona
Department of Emergency Medicine
Tucson, Arizona

N. Heramba Prasad, MD, FACEP
Associate Professor and Residency Director
Department of Emergency Medicine
SUNY Upstate Medical University
Syracuse, New York

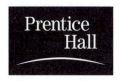

Prentice
Hall

Upper Saddle River, New Jersey 07458

Library of Congress Cataloging-in-Publication Data
Brown, Lawrence H., 1963–
   An introduction to EMS research / Lawrence H. Brown,
Elizabeth A. Criss, N. Heramba Prasad.
     p. cm.
    Includes bibliographical references and index.
    ISBN 0-13-018683-X
    1. Emergency medical services—Research—Methodology.
I. Criss, Elizabeth A.   II. Prasad, N. Heramba, 1947–
III. Title.

RA645.5 .B765 2001
362.18'07'2—dc21   2001046179

Publisher: Julie Alexander
Acquisitions Editor: Katrin Beacom
Editorial Assistant: Kierra Bloom
Marketing Manager: Tiffany Price
Product Information Manager: Rachele Triano
Production Management: North Market Street Graphics
Copy Editor: Stephanie Landis, North Market Street Graphics
Production Liaison: Alex Ivchenko
Director of Production and Manufacturing: Bruce Johnson
Managing Editor for Production: Patrick Walsh
Manufacturing Buyer: Pat Brown
Creative Director: Cheryl Asherman
Cover Design Coordinator: Maria Guiglielmo-Walsh
Composition: North Market Street Graphics
Text Printer/Binder: Maple Vail
Cover Printer: Phoenix Color Corporation

Pearson Education Ltd.
Pearson Education Australia, Pty . Ltd.
Pearson Education Singapore, Pte. Ltd.
Pearson Education North Asia, Ltd.
Pearson Education Canada, Ltd.
Pearson Educación de Mexico, S.A. de C.V.
Pearson Education—Japan
Pearson Education Malaysia, Pte. Ltd.

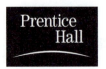
Prentice
Hall

10 9 8 7 6 5 4 3 2 1
ISBN 0-13-018683-X

DEDICATION

To my real mom, Carlyn Brown, and my EMS mom, Annice Peckham. Thanks for everything.—L.H.B.

To my family, Gary, Jason, and Sara, for all their support during the development of this project.—E.A.C.

To my wife, Barbara; my children, Michael, Yasmine, and Marissa; and my grandson, Dylan. I love you all very much.—N.H.P.

CONTENTS

SECTION 1   BASICS   1

SECTION 2   DECIDING WHAT TO STUDY   25

Chapter 13   Describing and Analyzing the Data   142

Chapter 14   Reporting the Findings   161

FOREWORD

The same issues transforming the health care delivery system in the United States are also reshaping EMS. Numerous issues affect our ability to properly assess the EMS System: The basic research models necessary to assess the EMS system are lacking; few EMS systems conduct significant volumes of research; and there are few academic centers that dedicate themselves to EMS research.

The perceived benefits of EMS have largely been based on historical precedent or anecdotes rather than on fact. In December 1997, Dr. Michael Callaham wrote in *Annals of Emergency Medicine,* "It is possible to document exactly how much scientific support there is for the efficacy of our present scope of EMS practice, and it is impressively deficient. There is virtually no aspect of EMS that could meet the current requirements of the Food and Drug Administration for approval as a safe and effective new therapy." Many in EMS took this as an insult and started to point fingers at other health care providers, implying that they too have not proven their worth. I saw Dr. Callaham's article as an opportunity to professionalize our industry. For EMS to be recognized, it needs to be respected. To be respected, we should justify why we are in existence and prove that we make a difference. Most of us feel that we make a difference, but can we prove it?

One of the largest barriers in research in EMS is the naïveté of the individuals involved in EMS, from the administrators and educators to the field providers and even some medical directors. Most EMS individuals have feared research, and because of this fear, it has been left for others to do. In some cases the individuals doing EMS research, although they had the best of intentions, used flawed research methodologies because they did not know the arena they were studying. In 1998 the U.S. Department of Transportation released the National Standard Curriculum for EMT-Paramedic. In this document, as never before, the authors of the curriculum included a section on research. Hopefully, in generations to come, as more and more EMS professionals learn about the process, research will become less feared and more accepted.

Developing EMS research disciples has been my dream. Having research included in the standard paramedic curricula is only a start. In 1992 a group of EMS researchers developed the Prehospital Care Research Forum. The Forum has a mission of assisting, recognizing, and disseminating prehospital care research conducted at all provider levels. One of the steps in pursuing this mission was to develop an

EMS research workshop. Today, more than 420 individuals have been educated through that workshop.

Until now, no text resources have been dedicated to educating individuals in the uniqueness of EMS research. I have known the authors of this text for many years. Collectively, they have extensive backgrounds in direct patient care, education, and research. They can back this up with over 100 peer-reviewed journal articles. Some of the authors were the original directors of the Prehospital Research Forum and participated in the development of the EMS Research Workshop. Between the three of them, they have likely educated more individuals about EMS research than anyone else has. Lawrence Brown, Elizabeth Criss, and Heramba Prasad are truly leaders in the field of EMS research.

I was delighted to be asked to review the contents of this text, and even more excited to discover the contents are in essence what could make the perfect EMS research disciple. The text is a perfect complement to any research course, but especially to EMS research workshops and courses. It is also the perfect resource guide for individuals who need that little refresher course. The authors have far exceeded my expectations in this text. The book is written in such a way that an individual can become familiar with research even without taking a formal course.

Much of the future of EMS will be determined by the changes that we are responsible for making today. We cannot repeat the mistakes of our past and continue to make decisions about EMS care, education, and systems design without careful evaluation of each existing and new innovation. I congratulate the authors of *An Introduction to EMS Research* for assisting us in controlling our own destiny.

—Baxter Larmon, PhD, MICP, Professor of Emergency Medicine and Director of the UCLA Center for Prehospital Care, Los Angeles, California

PREFACE

Many people never read the preface to a book. Having now written a book, we have a better understanding of the role of the preface. We'll probably read more of them; we hope you read this one.

This *will not* be the last research book you ever need to buy. Any one of the chapters in this book could, in and of itself, be the subject of an entire text. Some could be the subject for an entire college course, an entire semester of study, or even an entire graduate program.

This book is not designed to teach everybody everything that there is to know about EMS research. It is a primer, an introduction to the research process, particularly in our area of interest: EMS. While it is intended as a guide for the EMS professional—whether a field provider, educator, or administrator—who has an interest in research, it may also be useful to non-EMS individuals. This book is intended to provide a general understanding of the research process, to provide pearls of wisdom about and to identify pitfalls in EMS investigations, and to help the fledgling investigator begin the journey to becoming an EMS researcher. It is also designed to help experienced researchers—whether physicians, social scientists, basic scientists, or others—who are new to the realm of EMS research.

In writing this book, we struggled with our own grammatical shortcomings. We would have preferred to address you, the reader, directly: to tell you what you should do, how you should do it, and what to look out for. However, it must be recognized that appropriate grammar does not allow for the use of such a direct, personal approach. Thus, the authors have written this text in the distant but proper voice that one might find quite difficult to read. We're not very good at that, and we apologize in advance.

If you truly want to become an EMS researcher, there is at least one thing more important than buying and reading this book. You must have a good mentor. While this book can provide you with basic information about the research process and some insight into the world of EMS research, becoming a researcher is not an endeavor you should undertake alone. You would have never considered becoming an EMT by simply reading Brady's *Emergency Care* and then hitting the streets. You can't become a researcher that way, either. Finding a mentor isn't as hard as you might think, and it's one of the issues addressed in the appendixes of this book.

Welcome to the world of EMS research. It's been our home for many years, it's a great place, and we love it here. We hope you will, too.

—Lawrence, Liz, and Heramba

ACKNOWLEDGMENTS

We want to thank . . .

Dwayne Clayden, who first conceptualized and initiated the process of developing this text;

All of the reviewers, whose thoughtful and honest insights helped us to make this a better product;

Tracie Gardner, for reviewing the entire text from a non-EMS viewpoint and helping us to see its broader potential;

Stephanie Landis of North Market Street Graphics, for editing the final manuscript and making us seem literate;

Katrin Beacom, for bringing this project to fruition; Judy Streger, for getting us started in the first place; and all the people at Brady who helped to make this happen;

And Baxter Larmon, for writing the foreword to this text; for his mentorship; and—mostly—for his friendship.

REVIEWERS

Ann M. Fitton, EMT-P
New York City Fire Department
New York, NY

Guy H. Haskell, PhD, NREMT-P
Emergency Medical Services
Quinisigamund Community College
Worcester, MA

Linda Honeycutt, EMT-P, I/C
HealthStream/EMInet
Nashville, TN

Mary Kay Margolis, MHA, MPH
MEDTAP International, Inc.
Rockville, MD

ABOUT THE AUTHORS

Lawrence Brown, EMT-P began his career as a volunteer with the Perquimans County Rescue Squad in Hertford, North Carolina. In 1991 he joined the Department of Emergency Medicine at East Carolina University as an EMS instructor, and he quickly became involved in a number of research projects. Since then, getting EMS providers involved in research work has become one of his primary missions. In 1998 Lawrence moved to Syracuse, New York, where he spends too much time working and not enough time sailing.

Liz Criss, RN, CEN, MEd began her career as a research assistant in the Section of Emergency Medicine at the University of Arizona in 1983. She moved into prehospital research in 1984 and has devoted the last 17 years to prehospital research, education, and system development. In addition to prehospital research, she works with the Emergency Department of University Medical Center. Liz still lives in Arizona with her husband of 25 years, two grown children, her dogs, and a small flock of pink flamingos.

Heramba Prasad, MD, FACEP has had extensive EMS experience in three different states: Illinois, New York, and North Carolina. He has published a number of EMS-related papers and one previous textbook. In 1997, after 10 years as an academic emergency physician, Heramba took a brief hiatus to work in the community hospital setting. In 1999 he saw the error of his ways and moved to central New York, where he again practices academic emergency medicine, owns a horse farm, and claims to be a gentleman farmer.

SECTION 1

BASICS

Chapter 1

Why Do We Need EMS Research?

Medical research has been around for thousands of years. Five hundred years before the birth of Christ, Hippocrates discovered that an extract made from willow bark could be used to treat aches, pains, and fever. More than 2,000 years ago, ancient Egyptians determined that extracts made from the hibiscus flower were good for headaches. The extracts from willow bark and hibiscus contain a chemical called salicin. Salicin is the pharmacological forebearer of salicylates, which over the centuries became widely used for pain management. Through the years, physicians found that salicylates in their natural form caused significant stomach problems. So, about 100 years ago, a gentleman named Felix Hoffman set about finding a pain medicine for his father's arthritis that would not irritate the stomach. He synthesized a compound known as acetylsalicylic acid. His employer, Friedrich Bayer & Company, gave this compound the now-familiar name of aspirin.

A little more than 200 years ago, in 1775, England's Lord William Withering made a strange discovery: A poisonous plant called purple foxglove, which had been used for centuries in "witches' brews," had a peculiar effect on people. Some people, who were sick and dying, could be miraculously cured with purple foxglove. Other people, who were perfectly healthy, could be killed by it. It was only through careful observation and even more careful thought that Lord Withering finally figured out that the people helped by purple foxglove were those with congestive heart failure—those drowning in their own secretions. He further determined that it was people without any cardiovascular problems who died from its toxicity. Today we know the active substance in purple foxglove as digitalis—a drug that is still used to treat patients with heart disease, and one that can still be highly toxic.

About 150 years ago, in the mid-1840s, two physicians on two different continents made similar observations. Dr. Oliver Wendell Holmes noticed that there was a high prevalence of "childbed fever" in American hospitals. He believed that the infection was passed to pregnant women from the hands of their doctors. In Vienna, Dr. Ignaz Semmelweis observed that the mortality rate for pregnant women who were cared for by medical students was three times higher than the death rate for women whose babies were delivered by midwives. Seeing that the students were going straight from the autopsy room into the delivery room, he thought that students might be transmitting infections from their cadavers to their patients. Both

Holmes and Semmelweis recommended that physicians (and students) wash their hands—and both were ridiculed. It wasn't until 1865, when Joseph Lister finally proved that washing the hands with an antiseptic before performing an operation did indeed reduce infection rates, that hand-washing became a routine activity among physicians.

These are but three examples of medicines and practices that have become commonplace as a result of careful observation and research. But what do these examples have to do with EMS research? If medical research has been going on for thousands of years, why is there a need for more?

EMS IS DIFFERENT

Modern EMS can trace its beginnings to the pioneering physicians and spirited fire-fighters who undertook the challenge of moving the first 30 minutes of cardiac arrest management from the hospital to the patient's home. Since then, EMS has evolved to include prehospital care for many different medical and traumatic emergencies. Today, EMS is a multi-billion-dollar industry, but very few modern EMS practices have been subjected to scientific scrutiny. Instead, common hospital practices, equipment, and medical interventions have simply been adapted for prehospital use. The field of EMS, however, is unique. It defies the traditional hospital practice of medicine due to its less controlled environment and unique approach to patient care.

For centuries, medicine has been taught as an organized method of meticulously taking a complete and detailed history, performing a thorough examination, getting whatever tests are appropriate, and then formulating a treatment plan. This clearly will not work in the field of emergency medicine, and much less so in the field of EMS. In acute critical care situations, treatment is begun after a quick appraisal—the primary survey—and further evaluation proceeds concurrently with treatment. One cannot wait for all of the test results to come in when a lifesaving intervention is needed.

This unique nature of EMS medical practice, unfortunately, was not clearly understood in the early days of EMS. Because EMS was a new and emerging field, the people who wrote the original textbooks had very little knowledge of the EMS environment. It is not their fault; at that time nobody really knew what EMS was or what it would become. If something sounded reasonable, it was included in the teaching. Many hospital-based dogmas and beliefs were incorporated into EMS curricula, and many treatment approaches were advocated without validation of their effectiveness in the prehospital environment.

Eventually, the problems with this approach became clear. Now, after more than three decades of EMS, many of the teachings based on in-hospital care are finally being questioned and newer methods of providing patient care are being sought. Numerous examples exist of prehospital practices that lack a scientific basis. Research is now emerging that demonstrates the ineffectiveness or limited application of many of those practices.

UNPROVEN PRACTICES

Military anti-shock trousers (MAST) were once thought to be the most important piece of equipment on ambulances, able to save lives "with a single pump." About a decade ago, inserting an esophageal obturator airway (EOA) was considered appropriate advanced airway management. Even well-respected and established texts and classes advocated use of these treatment options, based solely on anecdotes and their intuitive value, but with no sound scientific evidence. Yet, now that they have finally undergone scientific evaluation, neither of these devices is widely used in EMS.

Today, there are new devices being touted as important tools for the EMS provider. Historically, EMS providers have been quick to accept new products—new gadgets—and incorporate them into their out-of-hospital practice. Instead, the process for new product introduction should include scientific evaluation of manufacturer claims. Testing these products before they become part of the standard of care is important. Not only does this practice save money, it also protects patients from potential harm. Rigorous evaluation in actual field conditions, including use by actual field providers, should be a mandatory part of all new product development.

EMS products are not the only area in need of research. There are also many examples of unsupported patient care interventions. Fluid resuscitation has long been a mainstay of trauma care, but researchers are now discovering that rapid resuscitation that restores blood pressure before bleeding is controlled may actually be detrimental in critically injured patients. The practice of elevating the blood pressure has been widely accepted because it seems like the right thing to do. It's what EMS professionals have been taught for years. Only now, however—30 years into the modern EMS era—are researchers finally scientifically exploring the best ways to manage the trauma patient.

Another example of evolving EMS interventions is in the management of poisonings. For many years, EMTs were taught to administer ipecac for ingestion of toxic materials. Today, the science suggests that ipecac is not effective at emptying the stomach, and is probably more risky than helpful. What was once the standard of care has been shown to be ineffective. Research is important not only for establishing the standard of care, but also for evaluating those dogmas that have become standards of care in the absence of evidence. Challenging the standard of care can be controversial and changing it can be difficult. All EMS practices, however, must be subjected to scientific research.

Does the lack of science in prehospital care mean that EMS should go back to "load and go" and not attempt any treatment at all? No. It simply means that EMS professionals need to explore all of the possible treatment measures, and find out what's best for patients; find out what does—and does not—work. EMS professionals need to do research. In 1983, Dr. Ron Stewart, himself a pioneer of EMS and EMS research, said, "If our methods and techniques are not changed to conform to what is medically needed, EMS as we know it will fade fast from the medical scene." EMS must develop its own scientific basis, its own foundation. It is not acceptable to simply rely upon research conducted in other fields of medicine.

THE STATE OF THE SCIENCE

A review of the medical literature from 1960 through 1999 reveals only about 5000 EMS-specific research studies. The subjects and types of studies reflect specific cycles in EMS history. In the mid-1960s, the first citations using the term *EMS* focused on disaster planning and response. In the 1970s, the emphasis shifted to cardiac care. By the 1980s, prehospital trauma care became the emphasis. During the 1990s, the literature began to reflect the general consensus that EMS may lack appropriate data to support its continuation.

A review of the literature also demonstrates an increasing number of individuals participating in EMS research, suggesting an increased interest in quantifying and qualifying the value of EMS systems. More and more often, individuals involved in out-of-hospital care are being listed as authors of studies.

Many EMS professionals have questions about things that are accepted as common EMS practice. All of those questions can be the basis for research. Is providing oxygen really dangerous to some patients? Is it true that patients in severe respiratory distress will not tolerate an oxygen face mask? Does every person in a motor vehicle crash have to be immobilized? Do seat belts really save lives? Do patients who have hypoglycemia that is successfully treated in the field need to be transported? What about asthma patients whose symptoms resolve? Does contacting medical control for every patient really improve patient care and outcomes? Do prewritten protocols enhance or hinder patient care?

These are but a few examples of the numerous questions about EMS that, so far, don't have good answers. While many EMS professionals are striving hard to find answers to some of these questions, more EMS professionals need to become involved in research in order to answer even more questions.

THE OTHER BENEFITS OF RESEARCH

There are other, nonclinical reasons to become involved in research. In order for EMS to be recognized as a separate specialty of its own, EMS personnel need to look at the field very closely and scrutinize every administrative, therapeutic, evaluative, and controversial issue. This is an area where a lesson can be learned from the experience of nursing. Since the early days of Florence Nightingale, many strides have been made to improve the professionalism of that specialty. It wasn't long ago that nurses were "there to carry out the doctor's orders, and not question them." They did not have autonomy or recognition for their expertise. That is no longer true. Through organized research, and application of the knowledge gained through research, the nursing profession has reached its present state of independence and recognition.

Another reason for pursuing research is simple economics. As funding for medical care becomes more competitive, patients and insurers are going to require that any services they pay for be proven effective. This can be a double-edged issue. If being transported by an ambulance doesn't improve the outcome for patients with wrist fractures, payers will start pushing those patients to go to the hospital by private vehicle. On the other hand, if hypoglycemic patients can safely be treated by paramedics and left at home, and that costs less than going to the hospital, payers will start pushing for EMS agencies to provide that service. In EMS, what does and does not work, and what is and is not cost-effective, is still an open question. Answering that question will help shape the future of prehospital care.

THE ROLE OF THE EMS PROFESSIONAL

Even if one accepts that research is important, an obvious question remains. There are people who are specially trained to do this work. Why should the average EMT or paramedic be concerned about doing research?

The first answer is that a person performing certain tasks, day in and day out, is in a unique position to discover problems and questions. Supervisors, administrators, educators, physicians, and others in leadership or academic positions may not recognize some of these issues. They may be even more unlikely to understand the importance of an issue or a problem, and they are not in the best position to suggest solutions. Like Hippocrates, Dr. Holmes, Dr. Semmelweis, and Mr. Hoffman, it is the person who is actually taking care of patients—in this case the EMS professional—who can best identify the truly important issues and help formulate possible solutions.

A second answer is that inquisitiveness is human nature. The learning process continues throughout our lives. That is how evolution occurs. Every EMS professional has questions. Every EMS professional wants answers. Becoming involved in the research process allows the individual to develop an organized method for finding those answers. That improves patient care, it improves the state of the profession, and it enables the EMS professional to become a partner in the evolution of EMS.

It's important to note that no one expects every EMS provider to become a researcher, just as no one expects every physician, every nurse, every engineer, or every biologist to become a researcher. However, all EMS providers are affected by research, and they must at least understand and appreciate its value. EMS providers who are not motivated to be researchers still play an important role in the research process. They can identify study questions, support research projects, and assist with data collection, and they must be open to the ever-changing nature of medical practice.

One might think, "I agree that research is important and I'd like to get involved, but I have no idea how to go about doing it. I don't know anything about research." In fact, almost every person feels some trepidation and hesitation on hearing the word *research*. Yet, without realizing it, most people take part in activities every day that qualify as research. Research is simply an organized attempt to find answers to the questions and problems that arise every day. Notice the word *attempt*. Research does not necessarily always result in a solution or a definite answer. Whenever an *attempt* is made to answer a question or solve a problem, research is being conducted.

The purpose of this book is to help EMS providers answer questions. For the nonresearcher, it teaches about the research process. For the EMS provider interested in conducting research, this book teaches how to get it done. Whether one is reading another person's research, helping out a colleague, collecting data for a systemwide project, or developing one's own question and research project, this book can help. It explores all the phases of a research project and includes a step-by-step process—a recipe—for conducting any study.

So what do the discoveries and experiments of Hippocrates, Holmes, Semmelweis, Withering, and Hoffman have to do with EMS research? Fifty, 100, or 1000 years from now, the EMS research that is done today will be viewed as the foundation—the ancient discoveries—upon which EMS practice is based. And the people who work in EMS today—those who ask the questions, those who do the research, and those who incorporate the findings—will be regarded as the pioneers of what become modern, scientifically based EMS practices.

Chapter 2

The Research Process

The goal of this chapter is to lay the foundation for conducting research projects. This chapter is an overview of the process; individual steps are more thoroughly discussed in subsequent chapters. By the end of this chapter, the EMS researcher should have a general understanding of the principles of medical research and the process for developing and implementing a research project.

RESEARCH IN LIFE AND MEDICINE

Research is life, and the research process begins at birth. Maybe *exploration, discovery,* and *learning* are better words, but it's all really the same thing. Babies put things in their mouths to figure out what they are, how they taste, and whether or not they like them. That's research! A 2-year-old learns the word *no,* and then tests his parents to see just how far he can go before getting a time-out. That's research! A 12-year-old starts sneaking a cuss word into conversations every now and then, just to test the limits of her parents. That's research! And the exploration continues throughout the life cycle.

The point is that everyone does research. Whether the research involves learning that a stove is hot or exploring the influence of genes on heart disease, the basic concepts of exploring, discovering, and learning remain constant.

The research that takes place during day-to-day living—just like EMS research—can take many forms. The two most common are experience and observation. Experiences and observations contribute significantly to a person's understanding of the world. Although they are not really perceived as "research," experiences and observations play a major role in the development of EMS practice, too.

Experience

Personal experience is also known as anecdotal experience. It is knowledge that is based on events or incidents that have happened. A real-life example is someone flinching when they hear a toilet flush while they're taking a shower. Although no scientific studies have ever proven that the water in the shower gets really hot if someone flushes a nearby toilet, it is widely known to be the case. Almost everyone has had the experience. MAST, or pneumatic anti-shock garments (PASG) provide an EMS example of anecdotal experience. Although most of the scientific papers about MAST question their value, there are hundreds of EMS providers who say, "I know they work, because I've seen them work."

Anecdotal experience is a reasonable source of knowledge, but anecdotes have specific strengths and weaknesses. One of the strengths of anecdotes is that they are real; they are actual experiences that someone has had, not just laboratory experiments in some unrealistic or controlled environment. They are believable, often logical, and maybe even personal. On the other hand, anecdotes are really just isolated experiences. It is impossible to determine if a given experience involves some cause-and-effect relationship between observations, or if the experience was simply a matter of good (or bad) luck. Anecdotes are not scientific; they are not objective. Still, a few personal experiences can sometimes overshadow all of the scientific evidence.

Nifedipine (Procardia) is an example of a medication that became completely unpopular after a series of anecdotes. For years, physicians and EMS providers treated hypertensive crises with nifedipine. One of the potential side effects—which was well known—was that nifedipine could lower blood pressure too much, too fast, and in an unpredictable manner. Then, in 1996, the *Journal of the American Medical Association* (*JAMA*) published a report on 16 patients who had bad outcomes after receiving nifedipine.[1] At least two patients died. That publication was the proverbial last straw for nifedipine use in emergency settings. A series of cases—anecdotes— became the basis for a widespread change in the standard of care for hypertensive crisis.

What's wrong with changing medical practice based on a series of observations or anecdotes? Anecdotes are not scientifically sound, and the nifedipine experience illustrates that as well as any. In a scientific study of the emergency use of nifedipine, the patient population would likely be controlled to include only patients with hypertensive crisis who did not have contraindications to nifedipine, the dose of nifedipine would be standardized for all patients, and an adverse reaction would be strictly defined. However, the 16 cases reported in the *JAMA* article included patients with presenting complaints of unstable angina and pregnancy-induced hypertension. Some patients received 10 mg of nifedipine, some received 20 mg, and some received 30 mg, and the adverse effects ranged from dizziness to death.

This is not a call to reinstate nifedipine as a first-line medication in the treatment of hypertension. Rapid lowering of the blood pressure is not recommended for hypertensive patients, and there are better medications for treating hypertensive crisis. The emphasis here is on the difference between anecdotal experience and research. While anecdotes—experiences—can be an excellent source for study ideas, they are not in and of themselves good science.

Observation

Observation is another kind of day-to-day research. Things that are seen or heard over and over again eventually become incorporated into what one understands of life. Many people learn the rules of a sport simply by watching it over and over again. With the exception of professional athletes, very few people actually study a sport and all of its intricacies. Yet, many people who have never taken a true lesson become able golfers, tennis players, or basketball players. Likewise, many EMS professionals develop practice habits based on their observations of other EMS providers or of emergency nurses and physicians. New EMTs and paramedics don't scientifically study the best way to interact with patients. Those habits develop by watching what others do. That is observational research: learning by observing what happens in the world.

Like anecdotal experience, observation has both strengths and weaknesses: Observations are real, clinically relevant, and sometimes personal. But, also like anecdotal experience, observations are often isolated, limited events. Any single observation may simply be due to bad—or good—luck. Any series of observations may be peculiar to a specific setting; things may be different in other places or in other EMS systems.

Observational studies differ from everyday casual observation in that they involve systematic observation. Observational studies can also be called descriptive studies. One example of a descriptive study was published in the March 1998 issue of *Annals of Emergency Medicine.*[2] The authors described 610 endotracheal intubations that were performed in one hospital emergency department. The study nicely detailed who performed the intubation, the success rate, the need to sedate or paralyze patients, and the complications that resulted from intubation. That kind of information could be very helpful to other emergency departments, and even to EMS systems that are starting to use endotracheal intubation.

What could be wrong with making decisions based on observations from another system? There's no guarantee that the actual experiences in other places will be the same as those described in an observational study. As with anecdotal experience, observations are not well controlled with specific patient populations and well-defined study criteria. For example, in the descriptive study reported in *Annals,* the decision to intubate was made at the physician's discretion, so the patients' conditions varied greatly. A resident often performed the intubation, and this study was completed before rapid-sequence induction for intubation became widely used. For those and other reasons, it may be hard to apply the findings—the observations—from that study to other settings.

Hypothesis Testing

So how does an EMS researcher—or any researcher, for that matter—avoid the perils and pitfalls of anecdotes and observations? By developing and testing a hypothesis.

What is a hypothesis? The dictionary defines it as "a supposition assumed as a basis of reasoning." It is really a researcher's idea, or best guess, about how things are. That's the tricky part about real research. The researcher doesn't just set out to find out, "What is the best medicine for cardiogenic shock?" The researcher has to make a guess—a supposition—based on his or her knowledge about the subject, and then test the accuracy of that supposition. A hypothesis would be, for example,

"Dopamine is better than dobutamine for treating people in cardiogenic shock." Then, the researcher would treat a group of people with cardiogenic shock, some with dopamine and some with dobutamine, and see if the dopamine really did work better. Testing a hypothesis is testing whether a supposition is accurate.

One EMS example of hypothesis testing is the supposition that vacuum splint backboards are less likely than traditional backboards to cause back pain in immobilized patients. The researcher doesn't ask if one or the other causes pain, but instead tests the supposition that one device causes less pain than the other. Chan et al. actually published a study about this in 1996.[3] They found that patients immobilized on traditional backboards were about three times more likely to report pain than patients immobilized on vacuum backboards. They tested the hypothesis; they tested their best guess—their supposition—about the differences between the devices.

The process of developing a hypothesis can be complicated. It is discussed in great detail in Chapter 5. In general, though, it is important that the hypothesis be specific and that the outcome be measurable. The biggest mistake most new researchers make is asking too big or too broad a question. To really answer a complex research question, it has to be broken down into little pieces, and each little piece must then be studied independently.

APPROACHES TO RESEARCH

There are several different approaches to conducting research. Primarily, the approaches are categorized by the types of data that are collected and by the methods used to collect the data. While specific study methodologies are discussed in Chapters 6 and 7 and an in-depth discussion of data appears in Chapters 12 and 13, a general characterization of these approaches is discussed here.

Quantitative vs. Qualitative

Quantitative data are measured numerically: How many? How much? How often? Is the average heart rate for a 16-year-old different from the average for a 35-year-old? How much blood will one 6- by 9-inch bandage absorb? Does 0.5 mg of epinephrine increase blood pressure more than 0.3 mg?

Quantitative research is objective and specific. A quantitative study might compare the exact heart rates of patients: 140 vs. 110 vs. 88 vs. 96 vs. 58 vs. 72. Those are exact numbers with exact differences between them. A qualitative study might describe those heart rates as fast vs. fast vs. normal vs. normal vs. slow vs. normal. Both approaches are accurate, but the quantitative approach is more specific.

However, it is often difficult to squeeze EMS issues into numerical form. How can patient satisfaction be measured numerically? How can EMT frustration be measured objectively? That's why qualitative research is important, too. It's less objective, less precise, and less numerical, but it allows the researcher to study questions that are not easily enumerated.

Because qualitative data are more subjective, they are measured descriptively: How good? How clean? How easy? A qualitative study might explore whether patients feel more confident with providers who wear uniforms. The researcher might ask the patients to rate their confidence on a scale from "none" to "extremely confident." Those are subjective, qualitative measurements. They are not specific, they are not exact: They are qualitative.

Although quantitative research is often regarded as more scientific, qualitative research plays an important role in EMS. Both types of research have strengths and weaknesses. Whether the researcher uses a quantitative or qualitative approach depends mostly on what he or she intends to study.

Prospective vs. Retrospective

In addition to determining whether a study is going to be quantitative or qualitative, the researcher also has to decide whether the project will be retrospective or prospective.

Retrospective studies look at information that already exists. Reviewing medical records, looking at old ambulance call reports, sorting through maintenance records, or gathering information from personnel files are some examples. Wherever they come from, the data in retrospective studies have already been collected for other reasons.

Retrospective studies are sometimes easier because the data already exist, reducing the time required to complete the data collection process. For example, if a researcher wants to compare success rates for IVs started on scene with those started in the ambulance, those data may already exist in the ambulance call reports. The researcher can spend a few hours, or maybe a few days, gathering all of the data needed to do the study. The downside of retrospective studies is that other people collected the data, for some other reason, sometimes a long time ago. Nobody was thinking about the current study when they collected the data, and some things that could be helpful to the researcher may not have been documented. In the IV example, it is possible that the EMT didn't specifically document whether the IV was started on scene or in the ambulance. It may be possible to figure it out by looking at the time the IV was started and comparing that to the time the ambulance left the scene, but those times are not always accurate. These types of problems almost always confound retrospective studies.

Prospective studies are studies that start now, examine what is happening now, and examine what happens from now on. Recording the respiratory rates, heart rates, and blood pressures of the next 73 asthma patients transported by an EMS service would be prospective. Distributing a survey at the next training meeting would be prospective.

If the study is conducted prospectively, the researcher can make sure everything that is needed gets recorded, can have it all recorded on one specific form, and can be assured that the same terms and measurements are used consistently. By using one specific form, the people collecting the data will know what is needed for the study, and maybe they'll be careful to be accurate and complete. In the study of

IV success rates, the form might include things like the type of emergency, the patient's age, the size of the IV catheter, where the IV was started, and the number of attempts. The downside of prospective studies is that they usually take more time than retrospective studies. In some systems, it may take 6 months or more to enroll enough patients to make the IV study worthwhile. If the researcher is studying a rare event, such as survival from cardiac arrest, it might take several years or more to conduct the study. Another problem with prospective studies is that the biases of the data collectors might affect the data.

As with quantitative and qualitative research, retrospective and prospective studies have strengths and weaknesses. These must be considered when determining which approach will be taken. As always, the approach depends on the research question, the type of data needed, the number of patients that need to be studied, and how much control is needed over the data collection process.

TYPES OF RESEARCH

In addition to deciding whether a study will involve prospective or retrospective data collection, and whether the study will involve qualitative or quantitative data, the researcher must decide on the type of study that will be conducted. There are three primary types of research: observational research, quasi-experimental research, and experimental research.

The type of study is dictated by how much, if any, control the researcher has over the intervention, or study factor. The intervention is the item being tested; the thing that might make a difference; the subject of the hypothesis. If a researcher is trying to determine whether 2 cups of sugar makes better iced tea than 1 cup of sugar, the amount of sugar is the study factor. If someone tries to determine whether 10 L per minute of oxygen is better for asthma patients than 15 L per minute, the amount of oxygen is the study factor.

Observational Research

At first, observational research might be confused with simple observation. The difference is that observational research is systematic in nature and tests a specific hypothesis; it measures the effect of some study factor on a specific outcome.

In observational research, the researcher does not control the study factor in any way. In a study comparing the test scores of older paramedics to those of younger paramedics, age is the study factor. The researcher does not control the study factor. He or she simply observes the difference between the two groups. The study could be retrospective (looking at past test performance). The study could be prospective (looking at performance on the next 10 exams). The study could be quantitative (measuring actual test scores). The study could be qualitative (asking students how confident they were in their answers). Independent of the basic approach, however, the study would be observational. The researcher is not controlling the study factor.

Observational research does have many of the same limitations associated with simple observation. It is more scientific because it tests a specific hypothesis, and because it looks at specific, predetermined data points. There is, however, still the potential problem that the system being observed may be very different from other systems. The study population may not be strictly defined and the study factor is not controlled. Since the study factor isn't controlled, there may be other factors that affect the results.

Yet, observational research does have a place among scientific studies. Almost all important epidemiological studies are observational studies. Most research on the risk factors for cancer and heart disease has been observational research. It would be impossible—and more important, unethical—to randomize people to be smokers, or overweight, or diabetic.

Quasi-Experimental Research

In quasi-experimental research, the investigator does control, or at least affect, the study factor. Quasi-experimental research differs from experimental research because the intervention in quasi-experimental research is not truly randomized.

If a researcher is testing the tea recipes mentioned earlier, and there are 18 pitchers of tea, he or she could put 1 cup of sugar in half of the pitchers and 2 cups in the other half. How does the researcher decide which pitchers get how much sugar? If that process is not completely random, then the study design is quasi-experimental. If 1 cup of sugar is put in every odd-numbered pitcher, and 2 cups in every even-numbered pitcher, that is not random; the study is quasi-experimental.

If an EMS study uses board splints for 3 months and then vacuum splints for the next 3 months, that is not random. The study is quasi-experimental. If the response times of two different EMS systems are compared—one system with system status management and the other without—that study is quasi-experimental. The project could be retrospective, prospective, quantitative, or qualitative, but it would still be quasi-experimental. The researcher is controlling the study factor, but not in a random way.

There is a reason why it is important to differentiate between quasi-experimental and true experimental research. When the study intervention is not allocated in a random fashion, there is always the risk of some systematic bias, or error, in the study. Perhaps a continuing education class on splinting was offered during the first week of the second half of the study comparing board and vacuum splints. That might affect the results. Perhaps the EMS agency using system status management has dedicated units for convalescent responses, while the other system sends the closest ambulance to all calls, whether emergency or convalescent. That could affect the results.

This does not mean that quasi-experimental studies are not valuable. In fact, a quasi-experimental approach may be the only reasonable way to conduct a study. It might not be possible—or at least practical—to randomly change the splints that are stocked on every ambulance. It would be impossible to randomize the use of system status management within an EMS system. Quasi-experimental studies play a significant role in EMS systems research and are often used to help formulate hypotheses for experimental studies.

Experimental Research

In experimental research, the researcher manipulates the intervention (the study factor), but in a completely random fashion. Randomization can be easy—simply flipping a coin is a reasonable way to randomize groups of two. Or the randomization can be sophisticated. Statistical texts usually contain randomization tables, and computers can randomize groups, too. However it is accomplished, randomization results in interventions being assigned simply by chance, without any direct influence by the researcher.

If a researcher is studying three drug doses, a randomization table could be used to determine ahead of time which patients receive which dose. There is no system to the allocation of doses; there is no sequence; there is no direct influence. Whether qualitative or quantitative, completely randomized projects are known as experimental research.

Bias can occur in truly randomized, experimental studies too. For example, the odds are that groups of patients randomized to receive three different drug doses will be roughly similar. By chance alone, one would expect the three groups to be about the same size, have about the same average age, and have the same proportion of males and females and the same history of risk factors. But because the process is truly random, without any control from the researcher, there's always a chance that the groups will be somehow different. If one of the groups, just by chance, ends up being 90 percent women, while the proportion of women in the other two groups is about 45 percent, that might affect the study results. Should a difference be found between the groups, there will always be a question as to whether the patients' sex had any influence on the outcome.

Some experimental studies try to limit the potential for bias by making the study population very specific. If three drug doses were studied only in men between the ages of 35 and 55 who had no risk factors for coronary disease and no history of recent surgery, the likelihood that the three groups would be similar would be increased. Unfortunately, the applicability of that study to other populations—women, older people, people with heart disease—would then be very limited.

THE EMS RESEARCH PROCESS

While the process for conducting a successful EMS research project can be thought of as distinct steps—sequential tasks, each to some extent building on the previous ones—it is possible, indeed likely, that many of the steps will be conducted simultaneously. Indeed, the problems encountered in any one step might also cause the researcher to go back and revisit a previous step. Each of these steps—each piece of the recipe—will be fully discussed in the following chapters. This section is designed as a template or resource guide that the researcher can refer to for each new project.

Choosing a Research Topic (See Chapter 3)

The research process begins with the identification of a topic for study. Once a topic has been chosen, it will then be reviewed and refined until it becomes a streamlined version of its former self. Novice and veteran researchers alike often begin the research process without thoroughly evaluating the complexity of their chosen topic. This is a very easy mistake to make, and one that can be easily avoided.

The researcher begins the process by determining an area of interest. EMS is one area of medicine that allows the researcher a broad base of possible topics. Studies can include all aspects of life, from its beginning through its natural or unnatural end. In general, EMS studies can be categorized as clinical, educational, or systems research. More specific topics include studies of how ambulance systems work, what systems work best for what types of patients, how EMS providers learn, or which splinting devices provide the most support and comfort.

These are all interesting topic areas; however, they are not focused enough to be considered for a research project. While the researcher may start with such a broad idea, he or she must then narrow the focus to a specific, researchable topic. Ultimately, the process should lead to an extremely focused idea.

Conducting a Literature Search (See Chapter 4)

A literature search is done to discover what research has already been done on a particular topic. The researcher may find many papers reporting on research ideas that are similar to his or her own. It's unlikely, however, that these previous studies will directly answer the researcher's exact question. Instead, these articles will help the researcher in refining the research idea, formulating a specific question and hypothesis, and designing the study. Even if a previous study has addressed the same (or a similar) question, that does not mean the researcher should not pursue the research. Medical science is based on several studies of the same issue—no one study should be considered as absolute proof of anything.

Most literature searches are conducted online using a computerized search engine. These are available through most major university Web sites, the National Library of Medicine Web site, and many commercial Web sites. These search engines use medical subject headings (MeSH headings, for short) to identify articles. *Emergency medical services* is a MeSH heading that will identify many EMS articles, but the indexing is not very exact. That MeSH heading will also identify emergency department studies, some disaster papers, and even emergency service communications articles. The researcher can also search for text words in the titles or abstracts of papers. This can help to weed out some of the articles identified by the MeSH search or to identify articles that don't exactly fit a particular MeSH heading. For example, the researcher could search for the text word *prehospital* and identify any papers that have that word in the title or abstract. Again, though, the indexing is not perfect. A paper titled "Pre-hospitalization insurance carrier approval for elective liposuction" would be identified by that search. For the researcher who is unfamiliar with online searching, the reference librarians at the local public, college, or university library can be extremely helpful. They're usually happy to help—it's what they do.

Another way to find relevant articles is to look at the bibliographies of other articles about the topic. If the research idea was generated while reading a particular paper, then review the bibliography of that article to see what references it lists. These papers will provide insight into the topic area, and they may also provide some guidance in structuring an online search. Review articles—articles that compile multiple references on a particular topic—are also very helpful in this way. These usually provide a list of current articles about the topic, as well as historical pieces that may help build the foundation for the study.

Developing a Question and Formulating a Hypothesis (See Chapter 5)

Generating the question and the hypothesis is the next step in the research process. The hypothesis is built from the question, and is a specific statement that the study tries to prove or disprove. The hypothesis states the results that the investigator expects to see at the conclusion of the study. The outcome is not actually known; it is just an educated guess made by the investigators. The formulation of the hypothesis is based on the researcher's question, personal experience, anecdotal reports, and the results of previous studies identified in the literature search.

The formulation of the hypothesis is another step in the research process where it may become evident that the proposed study topic is too broad. If it is not possible to develop a single-sentence statement that the study will either prove or disprove, the study question is probably too large. Words like *and, or,* and *because* should not appear in the hypothesis. If the hypothesis cannot be stated in a simple declarative sentence, then the researcher must reexamine the original topic and question, and then repeat the process of narrowing the focus. The goal of this step is to have a clearly defined, measurable endpoint. This is the crux of the project. Spending some time at the beginning to clearly define the hypothesis will prevent many common problems as the research process progresses.

Determining the Type of Study (See Chapter 6)

The type of study is influenced by a variety of factors, including resources, staffing, availability of data sources, and the type of question being asked.

Some of the different types of studies have already been discussed, and the process for choosing the type of study is more fully discussed in Chapters 6 and 7. Whether prospective or retrospective, whether quantitative or qualitative, and whether observational, quasi-experimental, or experimental, the selection of the study methodology will affect all of the other steps in the research process.

Developing the Methods (See Chapter 7)

The methodology of the study—the step-by-step process by which the study protocol is carried out—will be greatly influenced by the type of study. Developing the methodology for a study takes careful planning and logical thinking. The final product of this step should be the protocol or guideline to be followed during each phase of the research project. Serious consideration must be given to what data points are to be collected, where these data points will come from, who will collect the data, and when the data will be collected.

The methodology should be nitpicky, meticulous, and exact. The idea is to have a set of guidelines, a stepwise description of the research process, that everyone can follow exactly. The methodology for a clinical study will have to describe exactly how the experimental intervention will be made, on exactly which patients, and exactly what data will be collected. The methodology for a systems study will have to describe exactly how time intervals will be measured, or exactly how specific patient types will be identified, or exactly how cost estimates are calculated. The methodology for an educational study will have to exactly describe the curriculum for the program, or the testing materials, or the classroom environment. The devil is in the details.

It is important that the people who might be involved in helping with the study be asked to help with its design. They are the most familiar with their patient care process, their EMS system, or their EMS classes. If new data forms are needed, then set them up in such a way that it is easy for the data to be collected. Nobody likes to do more paperwork, so it's important to make the data collection process as easy as possible. This will also help with getting the researcher's colleagues to become partners in the project.

Performing a Power Calculation (See Chapter 8)

Because it is impossible to study every possible patient, or every possible paramedic student, or every possible EMS system, EMS research projects (like all research) depend on studying a smaller number of patients, students, or systems—a representative sample. Studying a sample, though, means the results of the study, whatever they are, will not be exact. The power calculation helps to determine how close to exact the study will be.

For example, a researcher might study the proportion of calls a system receives for diabetic emergencies. If the researcher reviews the calls for one year, the results might be that 13 percent of the calls in that year were for diabetic emergencies. That doesn't mean that 13 percent of all the calls the system ever received were for diabetic emergencies. The value for the previous year may have been 11 percent, for the next year it might be 12 percent, and for the lifetime of the system, the true proportion might be 9 percent or 15 percent. The more years the researcher studies, the closer to the exact answer the results will be.

The same is true for clinical or educational research: The more patients or students one studies, the more exact the results will be. Since it is not possible to study every patient or every student, the power calculation indicates how many subjects are needed for the study to be close enough to exact.

For most comparative studies, "close enough" means having an 80 percent chance of finding a difference between the groups if they really are different, and a 5 percent chance of finding a difference even if they really are not different. Put another way, "close enough" means the research findings could still be wrong somewhere between 5 percent and 20 percent of the time. A power calculation tells the researcher how many subjects must be enrolled to meet this level of accuracy.

The number of subjects needed—whether they are systems, patients, or students—is inversely related to the size of the difference one is trying to find and to the level of accuracy one wants to obtain. A highly accurate study looking for a very small difference requires a lot of subjects; a less accurate study looking for a larger difference requires fewer subjects. The exact number will depend on precisely what the researcher is studying, and will vary for each project.

Many EMS researchers omit this step, and their studies suffer for it. A study that does not have adequate power takes just as much work, just as much time, and just as much effort as any other study. The results of a study with inadequate power, however, are largely useless.

This is a step in which the researcher is well advised to consult a statistician. The process is described more completely in Chapter 8. Although it is a relatively small step in the research process, the power calculation is extremely important.

Obtaining Internal Review Board Approval (See Chapter 9)

Getting internal review board approval is also a very important step in the research process. Internal review boards (IRBs), also known as institutional review boards or ethical review boards, are designed to provide protection to the subjects that will be included in the research study. Internal review boards were established as a result of the atrocities committed by researchers in the mid-20th century. The IRB, composed of individuals representing medicine, sociology, psychology, theology, biology, ethics, and the general public, is tasked with conducting a detailed review of each and every project. Information submitted to the panel must explain how the study will increase present knowledge on the subject, how the patients are to be selected, and other pertinent issues like pain management and options for withdrawal from the study. Depending on the type of study, it may be necessary to inform the participants about the study and the possible risks, and to get their written, informed consent before including them.

Some studies are exempt from full review board examination. These usually involve review of existing data, specifically chart audits. Since no actual patients will be affected by the chart review, the panel can choose to exempt these studies as long as the investigator can provide the appropriate assurances that the patients' privacy will be protected. However, even when it seems obvious that no patient issues exist, the investigator cannot decide whether or not a study is exempt. The researcher must report the planned study to the review board and let that board decide whether it will require a full review process.

Most major publications require that authors sign a statement that the study has been reviewed and approved by the IRB, either fully or through the exemption process, before they will accept a manuscript for review. To find an internal review board, contact a college or university that participates in research, or the local hospital where the system medical director works. Each of these institutions must have a system in place to evaluate the actions of researchers or medical staff.

Interacting with Providers, Patients, and Physicians (See Chapter 10)

Most EMS studies cannot be accomplished by one person working alone. The researcher will almost always need the assistance—or at least the approval—of others with whom he or she works. A system study that involves the searching of records will require the approval of the system administrator and maybe the medical director. A clinical study enrolling actual patients will require the support and cooperation of the EMS providers working on the ambulances. An educational study will require the support and cooperation of the instructor and the students. It's important to get all of these people on board at the very beginning.

One of the best ways to get people to cooperate is to show them what's in it for them. For systems research, this could be notoriety, cost savings, or improved efficiency. For clinical research, it would likely be improved patient care, or better equipment. For educational research, it might be the learning experience of the research project or a positive change in the structure of the course. But remember, the researcher cannot guarantee what the results of the study will be, so be careful of making promises.

Once the researcher gains the support of colleagues, it is important to maintain that support. Most studies take time to complete, and people who are not directly involved in a project can lose interest quickly. Constant feedback and positive reinforcement are critical to keeping everyone on board.

Finally, give credit where credit is due. When the project is complete, the researcher should recognize everyone's support whenever the results are presented in any form. This will go a long way toward getting people to support and cooperate with future studies.

Conducting a Pilot Study (See Chapter 11)

The pilot study is an opportunity for the researcher to test his or her study design. While pilot studies are important, they can be difficult to do. For some studies, such as surveys or experimental trials, a pilot study may bias the final project by allowing participants to find out about the study prior to implementation. The positive side, however, is that the pilot study allows the researcher to find out what might be wrong with the design before it is too late to fix the problem.

A pilot study might reveal that a data collection point is not readily or consistently available. It might expose how long each chart audit will take. The pilot study might show that a survey question is misinterpreted by most of the people who read it, or it might show that field personnel don't comply with a randomization scheme.

No study design is perfect; taking time to conduct the pilot trial will reduce the number of problems encountered later on.

The findings from the pilot project should be used to make adjustments to the study methodology, to the data collection tool, or even—if necessary—to the hypothesis. It is much easier to correct these things earlier than to wait until midway through the study, when it will probably be too late.

Implementing the Study and Collecting Data (See Chapter 12)

This is the actual study, the stage where things begin to happen in real time. For some research, this will be the easiest part of the study. For other projects—particularly clinical studies—this will be the hardest part, the time when the researcher must be the most diligent about each and every aspect of the project.

If multiple individuals are collecting data, the data forms must be reviewed frequently to make sure all the data are being collected. Missing data can quickly damage a research project.

The researcher must also watch carefully for any unintended effects caused by the study or any component of the study. These must be recorded and, in some cases, reported to the internal review board or any funding agency. Some unintended effects may be serious enough to require that the study be stopped before data are fully collected. In most cases, however, this will not be a problem.

If data are being hand collected, it is helpful to stay current with the data entry process. Allowing too many forms to pile up before data entry will make the process more tedious and lend itself to errors in the database. Once data entry is complete, the data should be analyzed to document the rate of data entry errors. The statistician can assist in this process.

Analyzing the Data (See Chapter 13)

If a study is purely descriptive and doesn't involve any comparative analysis, this can be a relatively easy part of the process. Proportions and averages can be calculated and reported in their raw form. Sometimes, though, proportions and means are not the most appropriate descriptive statistics, and the researcher should be careful to report the appropriate results.

In comparative studies, the process of analyzing the data becomes more complex. An appropriate statistical test must be selected and applied to the data. There are many different statistical tests, and each has its own idiosyncrasies.

Ideally, the methods for reporting data and conducting statistical analysis are decided early in the research process, during the design of the methodology. A statistician—or at least someone with expertise in the area—should be involved in this process. Data analysis—sometimes even simple descriptive statistics—is not an area for the novice. While most researchers are capable of mastering the concepts, they almost always benefit from the assistance of an expert.

Reporting the Findings (See Chapter 14)

The final step in the research process is to report the study results. This can take a form as simple as a brief report to management about the implementation of a new protocol or as detailed as a manuscript submitted to a journal for publication. While each of these is designed for a different audience, the key components of each are the same.

A report of research findings should start with an introduction, including a brief history of the topic and the question/hypothesis being studied. Next should be a detailed summary of the methodology, including the approach to statistical analysis. The following section should contain the results, a factual presentation of what was found. It is often helpful to include charts and graphs in this section. Following the results, the researcher should provide a discussion about the ramifications of the findings.

SUMMARY

Research is life: exploring, discovering, and learning. Experience and observation play a major role in the learning process, and that is as true in EMS as anywhere. Learning through experience and observation, however, has limitations. To learn scientifically, researchers test hypotheses (their best guess—or supposition) about how things are.

Studies that test hypotheses can be quantitative, involving objective numerically measured data. They can also be qualitative, using more subjective data measurements. Such studies may be retrospective, looking at existing data, or prospective, evaluating data that are collected specifically for the purpose of the study.

There are three primary types of studies: observational studies, quasi-experimental studies, and experimental studies. The differences between these types of studies are related to how much control the researcher has over the allocation of the study factor. In an observational study, there is no control of the study factor. In a quasi-experimental study, there is some systematic control of the study factor. In an experimental study, the study factor is controlled by the researcher but in a completely random fashion.

There is no best approach or type of study. All of these approaches to research have strengths and weaknesses. The researcher must design the study in such a way that it will most effectively answer the specific question that is being studied. There will always be limitations and there will always be a chance of bias. While the researcher tries to limit these problems, they can never be eliminated.

The research process includes several steps, and the process for EMS research is no different. While some items in this process require more work, more time, or more effort than others, each is critical to the success of a research project.

SECTION 2

DECIDING WHAT TO STUDY

Chapter 3
Choosing a Research Topic

Choosing a topic is the first step in developing a research project. At first that might seem like a simple task, but it can, in fact, be very complicated. Everything that follows, from defining a question to reporting the findings, will be affected by the chosen topic. While the research process does follow a specific order—choosing a topic, then defining a question, formulating a hypothesis, and so on—each task should be undertaken with the understanding that it will influence all of the future tasks remaining in the project.

AREAS OF EMS RESEARCH

EMS presents a wide variety of potential research topics. As a young specialty, EMS is lacking a body of research unique to out-of-hospital issues. Most of what is incorporated into prehospital care practice is based on experience and observation. Since emergency medicine is the closest medical discipline to EMS, some practices are simply an extension of emergency department care into the out-of-hospital setting.

Almost all the potential EMS research topics can be placed into one of three main areas. Those three areas are (1) clinical research, (2) educational research, and (3) systems research. These are general categories, and many EMS research topics actually overlap into more than one area. For example, a study about an air medical program could be categorized as clinical or systems research; a study about EMT intubation could be clinical or educational research. As the topic becomes more and more focused, the category into which it best fits becomes clearer. Conversely, knowing whether one's interest is in clinical care, education, or system design will also help in the process of refining and narrowing the chosen topic.

Clinical Research

Clinical research is probably the area of greatest interest to EMS field providers. Clinical research focuses on taking care of patients: what works, what doesn't. This can include things like an evaluation of a specific drug, a therapeutic intervention, or a medical device. There are thousands, if not millions, of clinical topics that have never been fully explored in the uncontrolled prehospital environment.

Examples of topics that can be categorized as clinical research include the study of MAST, respiratory distress, or the treatment of hypoglycemic patients. In narrowing those topics, one might consider the effectiveness of MAST for blunt trauma patients in a rural environment. For respiratory distress, the researcher might wonder if albuterol alone is as effective as albuterol mixed with ipratroprium in adults with a history of COPD. Or, the researcher might explore whether hypoglycemic patients can safely be treated with glucose and then released by EMS providers. As the researcher moves closer and closer to defining an actual question, the topic becomes more specific.

Perhaps one of the most rewarding aspects of clinical research—its greatest positive attribute—is that the outcome can generate practical applications to benefit future patients. While educational research might measure how well students retain a skill and systems research might measure the impact of ambulance staging on response time, clinical research explores things directly related to patient care. That's not to say that skill retention and response times do not impact patient care, but their effects are often indirect.

The results of a clinical study can often be used to change clinical practice. Because clinical research can be directly translated into patient care, other EMS providers may be more likely to participate and to have respect for the findings. Educational and systems research can be perceived as bureaucratic endeavors, without true applicability to real-life patients. For the same reasons, EMS researchers might find greater satisfaction in conducting clinical research. EMS people like to believe that they have an impact on patient care.

Clinical research, however, can be the most difficult type of research to undertake. Particularly in the prehospital setting, the randomization and control of interventions needed for some studies can be complicated, if not impossible. In a clinical study, the researcher has to work with numerous other EMS providers and physicians who will be responsible for treating the patient and collecting data. Without their support and compliance with the research protocol, the study may take a longer time than planned to complete—or worse, may fail entirely. There may also be more ethical concerns associated with clinical research than with educational and systems research. When conducting clinical research, care must be taken to protect patient privacy during data collection and information storage. Care must also be taken to ensure that the study does not present any serious risk to the participating patients. Usually the patients must be informed of—and agree to participate in—the study.

Another difficulty with clinical studies is that the researcher must somehow balance and account for differences among the study patients, such as age, sex, preexisting conditions, or severity of illness or injury. If the researcher can collect data on a large number of subjects, it's possible that all of these variables will affect the two or three different experimental groups equally. If the number of patients is small, the potential effect of differences between groups increases. Variables that are not the focus of the research but that might still in some way affect the study results are known as *confounding variables,* or sometimes as *lurking variables.* If there are more older people in one group than in another, then that alone might explain a higher mortality rate; it might not have anything to do with whatever is being studied.

None of these challenges associated with clinical research is insurmountable.

The researcher who acknowledges that these issues exist can still design and implement a successful study. The trick is to recognize all the potential obstacles, plan for them in advance, and understand that there may still be a snag somewhere in the process. Accepting that no research project will ever be absolutely perfect will also help the researcher confront the difficulties of a clinical study.

Educational Research

At first, one might think that educational research would appeal only to EMS instructors. However, EMS education affects almost every aspect of prehospital care. While the direct impact of an educational program is on the students, there is a significant indirect impact on both clinical care and EMS systems. Education programs prepare EMS professionals to provide patient care and to function within EMS systems. EMS education programs affect everyone involved with EMS.

As is the case with clinical practice, very little research has been conducted in the area of EMS education. While education is generally a well-established and well-studied discipline, EMS education programs have developed mostly outside of traditional education systems. Even most community college–based programs are offered as extension programs taught by EMS professionals rather than professional educators, and they often do not adhere to the traditional education model. That's not a criticism of EMS education programs, only a recognition that most EMS education programs are different from traditional education programs. Thus, existing research about education may or may not be applicable to EMS education.

There are many approaches to EMS education research. A researcher may choose to study different methods of educating EMS providers: Is case-based learning really better than lectures? Are multiple choice tests better than essay questions? An EMS researcher might choose to study educational requirements: Is a 200-hour intermediate program better than a 100-hour program? Should paramedic students have to demonstrate a minimum reading level before entering the course? Finally, a researcher could choose to study how well students master a certain skill: Can basic EMTs learn to intubate? Do they retain the skill for at least 6 months? As with all research ideas, each of these can be further narrowed and refined, leading to a specific topic and ultimately a well-defined question.

One thing that makes research about EMS education attractive is that, so far, it hasn't received the attention other areas of EMS research have. A researcher with an interest in this area will find myriad potential topics that have never been explored. Another advantage is that EMS students provide an easily identified pool of study subjects. Because they are essentially a captive audience, it is easy to study students over the course of their education program. With the exception of those students who drop out of class, few subjects are ever lost to follow-up. Also, while there are ethical concerns that must be considered when using students as research subjects, including the need to obtain consent from the subjects, those concerns rarely include any risk of clinical harm to patients.

A particular advantage of EMS education research is that education in general has been widely studied. EMS researchers can glean ideas from these previous studies and take advantage of proven methodologies. If a researcher is interested in the relative value of multiple choice and essay questions, it is likely that previous non-EMS-related research on this topic will be identified during a literature search. The EMS researcher can often use the same methodology, or one that is very similar, to repeat the study among EMS students. This can be extremely helpful for the EMS researcher, since most EMS educators do not have formal training in educational research techniques.

On the other hand, the widespread acceptance of educational research principles and methodologies can also be a hindrance. Not all of the established educational research processes can be easily applied in the EMS education environment. For example, should an instructor who is exploring some classroom issue look for examples in the research involving community college students, technical training programs, medical education, or adult education? Or, is the accepted model for researching clinical internships in nursing applicable to the EMS field clinical experience? These are issues the researcher should be prepared to explore and address when developing a study about EMS education.

Another difficulty with educational research is demonstrating any clinical significance of the results. While test scores may improve with a given teaching method, that does not necessarily mean that patient care will improve. While students may prefer skills classes offered in 2-hour time blocks instead of 3-hour time blocks, that doesn't mean they're more likely to successfully perform a skill 6 months later. EMS providers, like most medical practitioners, often place great emphasis on clinical outcomes. The researcher must understand that EMS education research is about *education in the EMS environment,* and that educational outcomes are appropriate endpoints. The inability of the researcher's colleagues to accept that concept should not discourage someone interested in EMS education research.

One final limitation to most EMS education research is that the requirements for EMS education programs are not standardized. Programs vary from state to state, from community to community, and even from class to class within a community. Thus, the results of any single study might be hard to extrapolate to other education programs. This is true, however, for all three types of research: Clinical protocols also vary from system to system, and EMS system designs vary from community to community as well.

Systems Research

Systems research, on the surface, may be most appealing to administrative or supervisory people. But even the greenest rookie field provider has a stake in EMS system design. Every EMS provider, at some point, has wondered about his or her EMS system and thought, "Things would work so much better if only. . . ." Frequently, field providers and midlevel supervisors keep those thoughts to themselves, believing that upper-level management is not interested in their opinions or that the system is so burdened with bureaucracy that change is almost impossible. Often, upper-level supervisors and EMS administrators have the same "things would be better" thoughts, and *they* keep those thoughts to themselves because they don't believe that the county manager, corporate board, fire commissioner, or whoever they answer to, is interested in *their* opinion.

EMS systems research is an avenue through which anyone—from the EMT on the street to chief executive officer of a hospital system—can explore the potential for improving the delivery of prehospital care. It is the mechanism for testing those "things would be better" ideas. There is, of course, a difference between *studying* EMS systems and *changing* EMS systems, but EMS systems research can demonstrate the effects of system modifications and plant the seeds for change.

EMS systems research is also likely to overlap with the areas of clinical and educational research. Studies of ambulance staging might have some clinical impact on patients. Studies of employee retention might explore continuing education requirements or offerings. The extent to which a systems research topic extends into clinical or educational research depends mostly on what is measured. A study comparing the cost-effectiveness of two-paramedic crews to that of paramedic-EMT crews would be systems research. If that study measured on-scene times it would still be primarily a systems study, but on-scene times could be considered clinically relevant as well. If the study measured successful resuscitations, it might be perceived as a purely clinical study, although ambulance staffing is primarily a systems issue. Narrowing and refining the topic will make the distinction more clear, but systems research can be harder to isolate than clinical and educational research.

It might be easier, however, to develop ideas for systems research than for the other areas. Every "things would be better" thought is really the beginning of a research topic, and many of those thoughts involve systems issues. Other examples of systems research include studies that compare type II and type III ambulances, evaluate response times, explore fluctuations in call volumes, or measure public awareness about 911 use. Lights and sirens, air medical services, and expanded scope of practice are other topics that can be the subject of a systems research project.

One reason EMS systems research is important is because, to a large extent, it is the "basic science" of EMS research. The work that hematologists, physiologists, and other basic scientists do to figure out all the details of how our bodies work is essential to all of the other areas of medical research. Likewise, the details of how EMS systems work—and the best ways to measure and study those details—are essential to all of the other areas of EMS research. Figuring out how to make the system work better means figuring out how to take care of patients better. It's an indirect effect, but a real effect nonetheless.

Depending on the topic and the type of study, EMS systems research can be relatively easy to conduct. Systems often collect basic performance information that, although not intended for research purposes, can yield usable and valuable data. Call times, call volumes, patient characteristics, staffing levels, costs and charges, administered medications, equipment usage, and patient dispositions are just a few data elements that might be routinely recorded in an EMS system. Access to these data, particularly if they are maintained in a computerized database, can make for a quick, easy, and yet reasonably complete retrospective study. Another positive attribute of systems research is that it can usually be accomplished without involving every provider who works in the system. EMS administrators and supervisors often have a greater interest in EMS research, so the researcher might not have much difficulty in getting the support necessary to complete the project. Finally, since it might be easier to implement changes in a system than to change clinical practice guidelines, the researcher might gain more satisfaction conducting systems research.

There are negative aspects to systems research. It can be extremely difficult to control the many variables involved in a systems study. For example, how would one arrange to have some calls answered by ambulances housed at a fixed station and others answered by ambulances engaged in system status management? It can be done, but it can be difficult. It would be practically impossible to randomize those responses. Another limitation is that, as with educational programs, EMS systems are far from standardized and it may be difficult to apply the findings from one system to any other. Also, systems research is sometimes seen as a bureaucratic, meaningless exercise. Unfortunately, that belief is often reinforced when systems choose not to implement changes despite a study's results. This perception of bureaucracy, along with the problem of translating basic science research into tangible patient care activities, can be discouraging for the EMS providers working in a system, as well as for the EMS researcher.

SOURCES OF TOPICS

Choosing a research topic can be easy, or it can be frustrating. Sometimes the topic is clear from the beginning, usually when the researcher has a personal interest in a particular subject. These tend to be the best research topics, not because they are necessarily important issues, but because a researcher with a personal interest in a topic will work harder to complete the study. Working on someone else's idea, or an idea the researcher has no interest in, can be tedious. Pursuing one's own interest is exciting.

At other times, the experience of choosing a topic can be similar to writer's block or stage fright. Early in the process, when thinking about taking on a project, talking with co-workers, and even while reading this book, the researcher will likely have hundreds of fleeting thoughts about potential topics. But then, when it's time to actually choose a topic—time to write, time to go on stage—the researcher's mind goes blank. The few study ideas one can remember are immediately dismissed as too simple, too difficult, or of no practical value. Nothing "really good" comes to mind.

A solution to the writer's block experience—and a key to having topics available that are of personal interest to the researcher—is to keep a list of potential topics. Most EMS providers are constantly treating patients, talking with colleagues, attending classes, and reading EMS journals. All of those activities can generate questions that are potential EMS research ideas. The EMS researcher is well served by keeping a list of those ideas. The list doesn't have to be detailed, and it doesn't have to be well defined. The ideas can be as sketchy as "stroke/EMS" or as specific as, "Can EMTs identify stroke patients?" The researcher shouldn't spend time narrowing and refining topics when placing them on the list; that can be done later when that topic is actually chosen for study.

Before long, the list—which may become a complete file—will contain more study ideas than the researcher could ever possibly tackle. The list should be reviewed every few months, updated, and saved again. An idea should be removed only after the study has been completed—or when other researchers have sufficiently addressed the issue. Even if the researcher decides that the "stroke/EMS" topic isn't interesting, it shouldn't come off the list. Ideas that seem foolish today may seem like Nobel Prize material in 6 years. Old ideas will become the source of new studies.

For a new researcher who doesn't have a list, or for an experienced researcher who isn't excited about anything on his or her list, there are other sources for study ideas. As mentioned before, classroom experiences and patient contacts can be a great source for study ideas. Also, the researcher can talk with a system administrator or the medical director about things they'd like to see studied. Perhaps the best topics, however, come from colleagues—not from suggestions, but from complaints. Shift change meetings, dinner parties, company picnics, and other activities where EMS people congregate are a windfall for the EMS researcher. The things that EMS providers complain about, the things that they think should be changed, and their ideas for doing things better are all potential research topics. Those are also topics that the EMS providers will have a personal interest in, meaning the researcher will be more likely to have their support when conducting the study.

Another way to come up with topics is by brainstorming. The researcher can do this alone or with a group of colleagues. Start by simply writing down ideas. Again, these should not be too specific at this point; narrowing the topic comes later. This process is designed to just get the ideas on paper. It is effectively the same as making a list—it's just all done at one time.

A 30-second brainstorming session could produce a list of topics like:

Protocols
Documentation
Educational needs of students
Device manufacturer claims
New equipment
Air medical transport
Staffing
Medications
Critical care transport
Certificate vs. degree education programs
Respiratory distress
Seizures

Fluid resuscitation
Lights and sirens
Ambulance design
System status management
Prearrival instructions
Airway management

The researcher can start with these broad categories and then systematically narrow these ideas into topics that are ready for study.

FOCUSING THE RESEARCH TOPIC

Initially, one will probably take a broad approach to selecting a topic. A study of splinting techniques seems like a completely reasonable research topic. The difficulty, then, is narrowing the topic into one focused, well-defined issue. What aspect of splinting does one want to study? The researcher might then focus the topic to the effect of splinting on patient pain. While this is more focused, it is still too broad to study. Remember, the topic must be as specific as possible because even more specificity will be required when it is time to develop a question and formulate a hypothesis.

It may seem that narrowing the focus of the topic and making it more specific is the same as defining the question. While a focused, narrow topic does make it easier to define a question and formulate a hypothesis, that is an entirely different process. It is impossible to define a good question if the topic is not narrowly and clearly defined.

To continue with the splinting example, the topic might be further narrowed to the effect of padded board splints on the pain experienced by patients with broken arms. That's a reasonably focused topic, but it could still produce several questions and hypotheses. One question might be, "Do padded board splints reduce the pain experienced by patients with wrist deformity better than air splints?" Another question might be, "Does splinting a deformed wrist with a padded board splint reduce the pain experienced by patients with wrist injuries?"

The differences in those two questions may seem subtle, but they are in fact two very different questions. One compares outcome to determine if there is a difference between the two techniques; the other explores whether splinting with a padded board splint reduces pain. In fact, both questions could (and should) be even further refined. To do that, the topic must be further narrowed.

Continuously narrowing and refining the topic can be disheartening for the EMS researcher. It quickly becomes clear that one study, if narrow and refined, cannot answer an important question like, "Does EMS really make a difference?" All EMS researchers would like to have the answer to that question, but a study that attempts to answer it in one fell swoop is doomed to fail. The research process involves taking very small—narrow and refined—pieces of that question and forming each into a specific topic for study.

The process of defining a question and formulating a hypothesis will be discussed in great detail in Chapter 5, and the differentiation between these tasks, their interdependence, and their importance in the research process will become clearer.

SUMMARY

The first step in developing a research project is choosing a topic. Most EMS research projects can be classified as clinical research, educational research, or systems research. Many topics will overlap into two or all three of these classifications. All three areas of EMS research have both positive and negative attributes, no one area is better or worse than any other area. By understanding the advantages and disadvantages associated with each, the EMS researcher can design a study within these limitations that will be meaningful and successful.

Topics can be identified from many sources, including personal interests, patient care experiences, concerns and complaints raised by colleagues, and questions raised in journal articles or EMS courses. Brainstorming sessions are another excellent source for EMS research topics. It can be helpful to maintain a list of topic ideas, even though the researcher will never be able to actually study all of the items on the list.

Once a general topic is selected, the researcher must work to narrow the focus of that topic. A specific, well-defined research topic is essential in progressing through the next two steps: conducting a literature search, and defining a research question and developing a hypothesis.

A Typical Experience*
Part 1: Choosing a Research Topic

Tom and Mary were returning from the hospital after transporting a chest pain patient. They were talking about the chest pain treatment protocol, and how Tom—a paramedic for the past 17 years—always had trouble remembering to give aspirin. Even though the administration of four chewable baby aspirin had been in the chest pain protocol for quite some time, he still had to make a conscious effort to remember to give it.

"I guess you really can't teach an old dog new tricks," he said.

Mary, who had completed her paramedic training only 2 years ago, never had trouble with the protocol.

"It's just what I've always done, so I guess it comes automatically to me."

They talked for a bit longer, and both began to wonder whether other "older" paramedics had the same trouble that Tom did. They also began to wonder if it was really a big deal if someone forgot to give the aspirin.

*The characters and events described in the "A Typical Experience" sections of this book are entirely fictional. Any similarities to real individuals or events are purely coincidental.

"I mean, it's not like forgetting to give oxygen," Mary offered.

"Yeah, but it's still a protocol violation," Tom replied.

"I know, I know. But what I mean is, is it a big deal for the patient? Does it really affect their outcome? I mean, we know aspirin is a good thing and all, but does it make much difference if they get it in the ambulance or if they get it once they get to the hospital?"

"Well," Tom said, "it seems to me if something is important, then it just makes sense that the sooner you get it the better."

They were both quiet for a while as they rode down the highway headed to their post on the east side of town.

"You know," Tom finally broke the silence, "the other thing that bothers me is having to give those four individually wrapped pills. I always drop at least one of them on the floor when I tear the packaging open. You'd think they'd just give us a bottle, like they do with nitroglycerin. Or at least package them in fours."

Mary laughed. "Yeah, I've dropped a bunch of them too. I don't think the five-second rule applies when you drop a pill on the floor of an ambulance, but I've sure been tempted."

"What about when you drop it onto the sheet that's covering the patient?" Tom asked.

Mary hesitated, "Um, I think maybe I should take the fifth on that one."

"Nah," said Tom. "The floor is definitely out, but anything caught by the sheets is still usable in my book."

They arrived at their post, a gas station and convenience store at one of the major intersections on the east end, and both Mary and Tom went in to use the restroom and to get their complimentary fountain drink. Tom walked over to the aisle that had batteries, paper products, travel-sized toiletries, and over-the-counter drugs. He picked up a small bottle of baby aspirin and laughed.

"It's probably cheaper this way, too." For a split second he thought about buying the bottle, but decided that might not be the best idea.

Back in the ambulance Mary said, "You know Tom, they've got this new program where people who do research get priority when shift supervisor positions come open. You and I should do something with this aspirin stuff."

"Well, Mary," Tom said, "I've been here 17 years. If I wanted to be a supervisor, I'd be one by now. Why would I want that headache?"

Mary reached over and playfully punched Tom on the shoulder. "I wasn't thinking about you!"

"Oh, I get it," Tom smiled. "You know what, Mary? I don't think of myself as a research type of guy. But for you, I just might be willing to help out."

For the rest of the shift they talked about the possibilities. They came up with at least three possible study topics. They could do a clinical research project looking at whether giving aspirin in the field really made any difference for patients. They could do an educational study looking at whether older paramedics had more trouble than newer paramedics remembering that aspirin was part of the protocol. Or, they could do a systems study looking at whether using bottled baby aspirin was cheaper than individually wrapped pills.

"I guess we need to think about it some more," Mary said, "but if I had my druthers I guess I'd like to do a clinical study."

"Yep, me too," Tom agreed.

Chapter 4

Conducting a Literature Search

After choosing a research topic, the next step is to review the existing literature on the subject. The existing literature serves as the starting point from which the researcher can develop a thorough understanding of the problem, build a foundation for the importance of further research in the area, and formulate an appropriate study methodology. There are a variety of methods for finding reference materials and numerous sources for obtaining the literature. There are also some issues related to the strength and validity of the various types of information found during the search. All of these will be discussed in this chapter.

REASONS FOR CONDUCTING A LITERATURE SEARCH

The main purpose of the literature search is to discover what has already been published on a particular topic or topic area. The idea is for the researcher to gain as much knowledge as possible about the study subject before embarking on the research project. This will help the researcher to understand the problem, to convince others of the importance of more research into the issue, and to develop and design the most appropriate research methodology.

To better understand the chosen topic, the researcher must review the existing science about that topic. It is important for the researcher to have a solid, basic understanding of all of the issues surrounding a subject before proceeding. A researcher who intends to evaluate different splinting techniques for broken legs must know everything possible about both splinting and broken legs. A researcher who is planning to study the use of steroids for asthma patients must understand as much as possible about both asthma and steroids. It's not enough to simply review the existing literature about splinting broken legs or using steroids to treat asthma; the researcher's level of understanding must be much greater than that.

With a comprehensive understanding of the research topic, the investigator can begin to build the case for further research on that subject. The previous studies will have explored some of the issues surrounding a topic, proposed possible solutions, and revealed many shortcomings in the existing knowledge base. Even when those studies did not evaluate the specific aspects of the topics that are of interest to the investigator, they will provide insight into what further research is needed. If previous studies have explored the specific chosen research topic, they may still indicate a need for further study. Changes in clinical practice, teaching methods, or system design should never be based on one single study—there's always a way to improve the study protocol or refine the study question and further validate the findings. Having a thorough understanding of the existing literature will help the researcher to determine the next logical step in evaluating the subject.

While determining the study methodology is a distinct step that comes later in the research process, it must be kept in mind when reviewing the literature, defining the research question, and developing the study hypothesis. As part of the literature review, it is important to evaluate the way others have handled studies on the chosen topic. Survey tools, scoring mechanisms, intervention techniques, and analytical approaches are only a few of the useful things a researcher might find in the existing literature.

Another reason for reviewing the literature is to avoid "reinventing the wheel." There is no need to experience all the difficulties, discoveries, problems, and mistakes associated with a particular methodology if someone else has already done that. A well-written research article will point out the limitations and the problems that were encountered during the study, describe how the investigators dealt with those issues, or suggest alternatives for future studies. Such information is usually found in the "Discussion" or "Limitations" section of the article. These sections of the article should be read very carefully; valuable information about future project development is contained here. The smart researcher learns from the mistakes of others!

Becoming an expert on the study topic will provide benefits in every subsequent step of the research process. Keeping the data collectors motivated about the research project, keeping management or other interested people posted on the progress of the project, convincing the internal review board (IRB) to approve the project, and working with the statistician on the analysis will all be much easier if the researcher knows the subject well. A thorough knowledge of the existing literature also makes the preparation of the final report or manuscript easier.

MECHANISMS FOR FINDING THE MATERIALS

There are three main ways to identify the literature needed for a research study: self-conducted computerized searches, consulting a reference librarian, and personal reading. Each of these approaches has both positive and negative attributes, some that speed the process along and others that require a great deal of attention and detail. Most researchers will use all three techniques. Remember, the goal is to develop a comprehensive understanding of the published research available on the particular research topic.

Certainly the most frequently used of the three methods is computerized searching. Most major university-based libraries, hospital libraries, and public libraries possess computer systems that can search the literature with the use of key words or phrases. These libraries are connected to an online service that provides access to reference databases such as Index Medicus. Index Medicus is the most widely accepted and comprehensive resource for locating peer-reviewed publications. Updated monthly, Index Medicus provides a listing of articles from most major research-based medical journals. Index Medicus evaluates research journals before including them in the database to verify that they publish scientifically sound papers. Other searchable databases include the Cumulative Index to Nursing and Allied Health Literature (CINAHL), Educational Resources Information Center (ERIC), and Health and Psychological Instruments (HAPI). These are only a few examples; there are more than 50 searchable online databases.

These databases allow the researcher to search for articles in many ways. Medical subject headings (MeSH headings) and key words are the most common search mechanisms, but the databases can also be searched by journal title, author's name, or year of publication. The available search fields vary a little from database to database, but they are all generally similar.

Once an article is identified, it is usually possible to view an abstract (an abbreviated summary of the article) in order to decide if the article is related to the research topic and/or merits further reading. If the article could be useful, then the researcher can usually print the relevant reference information directly from the screen. This printout will contain all the information needed to locate the article on the library shelves, including the author's name, the title, the journal name, the journal volume number, and the page numbers. However, it may not be necessary to have access to a library to be able to obtain the articles. Some Web sites provide online access to journals, either free or for a small fee. Once access to these sites is obtained, the articles can be downloaded directly to a printer.

The second way of identifying research is to work with a reference librarian. Although online searching has made it easy for researchers to explore the literature without the aid of a reference librarian, it is still important for researchers, especially those new to the process, to discuss their search strategy and research plans with a librarian before attempting a literature search. Librarians remain (and should remain) the number one source for finding reference materials. These men and women are specially trained in the latest techniques for conducting literature searches, and are the most experienced searchers one can find. Articles are indexed by the MeSH headings, and librarians are particularly skilled at using these to find relevant articles. They can frequently find publications that even the most experienced researcher may not find on his or her own. Equally important is that remote places that are not near a major university or health sciences complex may find it hard to locate a specific journal or article. The librarian can assist in getting a copy of the article from another library, or may provide guidance in using a Web site to download the manuscript.

The third way to find relevant articles is through personal reading. A researcher should routinely read as many of the journals related to the field of interest as possible. For the new researcher, reading published literature is an excellent way to learn about various research methodologies and their application in the out-of-hospital arena. Reading will also help the researcher to gain expertise on many topics, and to obtain a general sense of current research trends. The researcher will also come across specific articles that relate to both the current and potential future research subjects. The reference list of any such journal article will provide instant access to even more material relevant to that subject matter. Reading those articles, especially if the article is on a similar topic, can also help provide direction for developing a more comprehensive literature search. Review articles—specialty articles that discuss and interpret all the relevant literature related to a specific topic—are an excellent resource both for obtaining information and for identifying other references.

CONDUCTING THE SEARCH

To fulfill the goals of the literature search, the researcher must perform the most comprehensive review possible. Working with a librarian is the best way to ensure that the literature search is all-inclusive, but for researchers who choose to do their own online searching, the following are some basic strategies.

When developing the search strategy, be sure to carefully consider how far back to search the literature. The online databases can go back as far as the 1960s, and references found in those early papers may date back as far as the 1940s and 1950s. Sometimes a researcher can find historical citations dating back centuries. EMS, however, is a particularly young area and it may not be necessary to search the older literature. From a practical perspective, the older citations may be interesting, but they are less likely than recent studies to contribute to the researcher's understanding of a given topic.

Begin the literature search by querying the information database with MeSH headings, key words, or phrases that are general in nature. Starting out with search terms that are too specific reduces the number of articles identified, potentially missing important articles not listed under those specific key words or phrases. It will probably be necessary to search several headings, key words, and phrases. Also, each MeSH heading, or MeSH term, can incorporate several subterms. The researcher can include these in the search strategy by "exploding" the MeSH term. This effectively casts a broad net, identifying as many papers as possible. The librarian can help with this process.

Initiating a literature search in this sweeping fashion is the best way to capture all of the articles about a specific topic. This can be particularly important when the topic is new or innovative because the indexing of such papers is often inconsistent. This is most likely to occur when the research topic is a new piece of equipment or a new treatment modality. In such cases, it may be necessary to look at articles dealing with similar topics in an inpatient or hospital setting, or to read papers on the same general topic that look at other specific issues. One example of this might be a literature review concerning a new type of immobilization device. If the device uses a new, unique method of immobilization, then a researcher would not expect to find any literature addressing that specific technique. However, a comprehensive literature search might reveal 30 or 40 articles evaluating other immobilization devices, some that might be similar as well as some that might be very different. This gives the researcher an opportunity to compare and contrast each article, to determine how the new immobilization technique might compare to the previously studied techniques, and to find strengths and weaknesses in the study methodologies that can be taken into consideration when developing the methods for the current study.

One important thing to remember when searching the literature is that the subject heading *emergency medical services* is not constrained to prehospital care. It refers to the broader concept of EMS systems and includes subterms like emergency communications, emergency psychiatric services, and hospital emergency care. The terms *ambulances* and *transportation of patients* are often more successful at identifying papers about prehospital care.

From the results of these initial queries, the researcher can begin to narrow the search to identify the most relevant topics. The most common techniques for doing this are combining and limiting sets.

If the first search included the terms *oxygen* and *asthma,* the results would be every paper about oxygen and every paper about asthma. The investigator can combine those two sets to identify those papers about oxygen *and* asthma. Or, if the search terms return two sets of papers on similar topics, the researcher may want to identify all of the articles in either set. For example, if the researcher is interested in surgical airways, the search terms *cricothyroidotomy* and *tracheotomy* can be entered. The search engine can then form a set of cricothyroidotomy *or* tracheotomy, which would contain every paper in either set but remove any duplicates.

Every search engine works a little differently, and the investigator has to be careful when combining sets using terms like *and, or,* and *not.* Table 4.1 shows six actual examples of searches with only small differences in the search strategy. The results, however, differ greatly. All of these nuances are supporting arguments for involving a librarian in the literature search process.

Limiting sets is also a way to discard those papers that the researcher knows in advance will not fit the research topic. The search results can be limited by the type of study, the type of subjects, the type of journal, the age of the subjects, and the language of the literature. For example, limiting the results to *human studies* will discard all of the laboratory and animal studies. Limiting the results to *most recent update* will discard everything except for the newest research. Limiting the results to *age greater than 18* will eliminate all of the pediatric research. While limiting sets is an easy way to reduce the number of citations identified, the researcher must be cautious when doing this. Again, the idea is to become as knowledgeable as possible about the topic, and understanding all of the research about a topic is an important part of the process. There might be results from animal trials or pediatric trials that could be helpful to the researcher even when the planned study involves adult humans.

Once the researcher has narrowed the search by combining MeSH headings, key words, and key phrases, and by limiting the results, the next step is to review those results and make some cursory judgement about the appropriateness of the articles. All of the online search engines will provide a list of titles, and most will enable the searcher to view an abstract from the paper. Beware: making a judgment about a paper based on its title or its abstract is a dangerous practice. At this early stage it is

Table 4.1   Index Medicus Searches Using Medline, 1997–2000

TERM	NUMBER OF CITATIONS
SEARCH 1	
1. Cerebrovascular accident	887
2. Emergency medical services	1776
3. 1 *and* 2	4
SEARCH 2	
1. Cerebrovascular accident	887
2. Emergency medical services	1776
3. 1 *or* 2	2659
SEARCH 3	
1. Cerebrovascular accident	887
2. Emergency medical services	1776
3. 1 *not* 2	883
SEARCH 4	
1. Cerebrovascular accident (explode)	3089
2. Emergency medical services (explode)	5452
3. 1 *and* 2	19
SEARCH 5	
1. Cerebrovascular accident (explode)	3089
2. Emergency medical services (explode)	5452
3. 1 *or* 2	8522
SEARCH 6	
1. Cerebrovascular accident (explode)	3089
2. Emergency medical services (explode)	5452
3. 1 *not* 2	3070

better to have a low threshold for inclusion. Unless it is absolutely clear that a paper is not related to the topic of interest, the best bet is to keep the article on the list and get a copy of the entire paper. Titles and abstracts are, in effect, the advertisement—the hook—for the paper. To truly judge the value of any paper, the researcher must read the entire paper.

Inevitably, the researcher will find that a first attempt at the literature search doesn't identify as much information as he or she hoped it would, and so the process is repeated. The search strategy is revised, another broad net of terms is searched, those results are refined through the combination and limitation of sets, those titles and abstracts are scanned, and those papers that address the chosen topic are identified. With the help of a librarian, it may be possible to complete a search in 2 or 3 passes; without help, a researcher may be able to perform a comprehensive search in 5, 8, or maybe 10 passes. Get the message: Use a librarian!

OBTAINING THE ARTICLES

Identifying the articles is just the first step in the literature review process. Next, the researcher must locate and read the articles. If the researcher has access to a medical library, most of the references will probably be available there. When going to the library to find the identified articles, it is important to remember that the printed citations included in computerized databases, books, and other journal articles can contain errors. During the printing and publication process, it is not uncommon for numbers or letters to be accidentally transposed, significantly altering the citation. Common errors include incorrect volume or issue numbers, transposition of page numbers, erroneous publication data, or misspelling of an author's name. While it is possible to find an article with just the (correct) journal title, volume number, and page numbers, the wise researcher will go to the library with as much information as possible. This way, if one of the pieces of information is incorrect, it will still be possible to locate the article using the remaining information.

Obtaining the actual articles can be expensive. At 5 cents per page, copying 100 articles that average six pages each will cost $30. One way to reduce these costs is to plan to spend several hours at the library. By reading—or at least scanning—the articles at the library, the researcher can further narrow the results of the literature search and only copy those articles that will be needed for future reference. If an article is not available at the local library and the researcher believes the article may be particularly valuable, it is possible to request a copy through an interlibrary loan. There is a fee for this, so use it wisely.

There are sources other than medical libraries for obtaining journal articles, but they are typically less reliable and less complete. The researcher might subscribe to one or more emergency medicine or EMS-related journals, and can access the articles in those journals directly. The researcher's colleagues, the system medical director, or other local physicians might subscribe to other relevant journals, and the investigator may be able to borrow some of those. The researcher can also purchase a single copy of a particular journal issue from the publisher, but that's usually quite expensive.

The most direct approach to obtaining a paper that isn't available at the library is to write to the author of the paper and request a copy. Most authors are interested in discussing their work and will usually share openly the various components of their project. This can be particularly helpful if an article mentions a specific evaluation tool or piece of monitoring equipment that might be applicable to the researcher's current project. The only time this might become difficult would be if the evaluation tool were proprietary and the author owned the rights to its future use. In this situation, many authors would still allow other researchers to use the tool, but would require some acknowledgement that the tool was developed by and is the property of the original author. Some authors might charge a fee.

A growing source for obtaining copies of journal articles is the Internet. Many journals make full text versions of their articles available online, and a large number of these can be accessed for free. Indeed, some of the search engines provide links that take the researcher directly to the online version of the manuscript. Unfortunately, these online full text articles are usually limited to relatively recent publications, and not all journals participate. Still, this is a useful resource, and its popularity is continuously growing. Some researchers believe that online full text versions of manuscripts will someday become the primary source for reference material, replacing traditional medical libraries.

ISSUES RELATED TO RESEARCH LITERATURE

The literature identified through the search process can come from a variety of places and can be in several different forms. As important as it is to know how to obtain a listing of pertinent citations, it is equally important to know which of the citations is the most scientifically sound and most appropriate for review in developing a research project. Not all literature is created equal. There are several types of articles that can be identified during a literature search. Full research manuscripts report all aspects of a research project. These are the most complete reports of a project and, customarily, what the researcher cites in a bibliography. A literature search may also identify preliminary reports, case reports, trade magazine articles, textbooks, Web sites, letters to the editor, editorials, abstracts, and review articles.

The primary source for research-based literature is peer-reviewed journals. These are usually specialty-based journals that publish original research conducted by members of that specialty. There are emergency medicine journals, surgery journals, pediatric journals, cardiology journals, and even a few EMS-specific journals. A literature search on an EMS-related topic likely will reveal articles from all of these and many other journals. The important thing to remember is that peer-reviewed (also called refereed) journals have the highest standards for publication. The studies published in these journals are subjected to review by other researchers to ensure their validity before they are published.

Preliminary reports are sometimes published in the peer-reviewed literature, but the researcher must be careful to remember that the results are, indeed, preliminary. Such studies are usually constrained by a small sample size, too broad a question, or an unproven methodology. These reports can be useful in establishing the importance of a problem and in designing the methodology for future studies, but by their nature the results of such reports should be considered inconclusive.

Case reports, or case series, are simply reports of anecdotal experience. While such articles usually include a review of the literature concerning the topic at hand, they do not represent science in their own right. Again, these papers can be used to establish the scope of a problem and as background information for future studies, but in and of themselves they do not represent research.

Articles published in trade magazines may be valuable, but they are usually not subjected to rigorous scientific review. While many trade journals do incorporate a review process, that process is less stringent than that of scientific peer-reviewed journals and is usually more of an editorial review than a scientific review. Articles in trade publications usually do not contribute to scientific understanding of a given topic, and are rarely helpful in designing a study methodology. Still, information from trade journal articles can be useful in describing a particular problem and the approaches others have taken to address the issue.

Textbooks can be another useful source for material about a specific topic. While the information in most textbooks is several years old by the time the book becomes widely available, the information is usually accurate and can help the researcher develop a greater understanding of a specific topic. Also, the research cited in the bibliography of a specific book chapter might be useful to the investigator, and might help the researcher identify other reference articles. Further, the author of the chapter may specialize in that topic, and the researcher could then search Index Medicus using the "author's name" field to identify even more articles.

The Internet is a new and evolving source for information. It is nearly impossible, however, to determine if the information retrieved from any given Web site is accurate. When using the Internet as an information resource, be sure to use only those sites associated with the U.S. government, major universities, or well-known organizations like the American Heart Association, the American Cancer Society, or other established professional organizations. These Web sites carefully screen the information contained on their pages for accuracy and authenticity. Be forewarned, though, that Web sites are dynamic, and the information found on a particular site today may not be there next week, next month, or next year. If having future access to the information contained on a Web page is important, the researcher is well advised to download or print the information.

Letters to the editor or editorials usually have little value in the development of a research project. They may provide good background material; however, they are biased from the viewpoint of the author or the journal. Some journals do publish brief research papers under the heading of "Letters" or "Correspondence." In these situations the information may be more scientific, but there is a reason the information is not published as a research article. At best, the contents of these articles should be considered equivalent to preliminary reports or case reports.

The abstracts of the research projects presented at many major research conferences are often published in peer-reviewed or trade journals. Abstracts present a snapshot view of the research and the findings. These short summaries usually lack complete detail. Relying solely on the abstract of a research project can be very misleading. If the research is relatively recent, it is possible that the author has completed a full-fledged manuscript that has yet to complete the review process and be published. In that case the researcher may want to contact the author of the abstract to gain more information. If the abstract is several years old and no complete paper on the study has been published, the researcher should be even more skeptical of the value of the study. Again, it may be useful to establish a foundation for future research or to describe a problem, but an abstract alone should not be the basis for a study methodology, a particular intervention, or an approach to analysis.

The researcher should be pleased to find a review article on the chosen research topic. A review article is a comprehensive examination of all of the literature about a particular topic. Review articles are extremely helpful to the researcher trying to develop a complete understanding of a particular issue. An investigator can often identify many worthwhile reference articles from the bibliography of a review article.

INTERNATIONAL AND FOREIGN-LANGUAGE ARTICLES

One final issue of importance is the country of origin of the research. A thorough literature search, especially one in which a language was not specified during the search phase, will reveal numerous articles originating from other countries. These may provide interesting reading, but the findings and methodologies may or may not prove useful. While the pathophysiology of humans is the same all over the world, there are significant differences in the way EMS systems operate in different countries and cultures. The researcher should read articles from other countries carefully to determine how the methods and the results might be affected by differences in cultures and medical systems. Sometimes foreign papers are extremely useful; other times they add little to the development of a project.

If the paper was originally published in a foreign language, that can create great problems for the investigator. Most search engines can provide an abstract that has been translated into English, but the entire article is usually not translated. The investigator must decide, based on the information in the abstract, if it will be helpful to obtain an English-language version of the paper. Libraries and universities can sometimes help with obtaining translated versions of a manuscript, but not all can deal with all languages. Inevitably, most researchers omit foreign-language articles as a matter of convenience. It's a practical reality that, unfortunately, shortchanges the scientific process.

SUMMARY

Conducting a literature search is one of the most important aspects of developing a research project. It provides excellent background material for the research project, an opportunity to see what has already been done on the topic, and a source by which the researcher can evaluate various study methodologies. Computerized search engines are the most common method used to identify reference materials, but even the most experienced investigator can benefit from the assistance of a research librarian when conducting a literature search.

There are a variety of sources from which research papers can be obtained, the most common being peer-reviewed journals. The mission of these journals is to provide a forum for researchers to publish findings gleaned from original research. Other members of the medical community evaluate the articles before they are accepted for publication. While this reduces the likelihood of an article of poor quality being published, it is not a guarantee. Other sources for articles can include trade journals, textbooks, or Web sites on the Internet. The relative value of each of these sources varies, but ultimately it's the responsibility of the investigator to review each piece of literature and determine its value to any given research project.

A Typical Experience
Part 2: Conducting the Literature Search

"Hey Tom, look at all these articles I've got." Mary plopped a pile of photocopies onto the station house table, where Tom was finishing off the last bits of a sausage biscuit and a cup of black coffee.

"What's all this?" he asked.

"It's for the chest pain and aspirin study," she replied. "I went to the library over at the medical school, and the guy there helped me find these."

Tom laughed aloud. "You spent your two days off in the library working on this? I'd already almost forgotten about the whole idea."

Mary frowned. "So now you don't want to help with this?"

"I didn't say that. I guess I just didn't expect you to get so carried away." Tom cleared away his napkin and empty Styrofoam coffee cup, let out a long sigh, and said, "Well, show me what you've got."

"So here's the search strategy we used," Mary began. "Since we were at the library we were able to search using Ovid, but the guy said I could have done the same thing using PubMed from my computer at home. First we used the MeSH heading *aspirin* and exploded that, and then we also exploded *emergency medical services*."

"Whoa," Tom interrupted, "what do you mean, exploded?"

"Oh, that just means looking at all of the articles that are indexed by that term, or any of the subcategories under that term. I can show you how it works on the computer if you want, but basically it's a way of making sure you get anything and everything even remotely related to whatever you're searching for—in our case aspirin and EMS."

"OK, continue." Tom began leafing through the photocopies.

"So anyway, of course using terms like aspirin and EMS gave us almost 100,000 papers, but then when we just got the ones that were about both aspirin *and* EMS, there were only 29."

"Wow." Tom was impressed. "There's already been 29 other studies about EMS giving aspirin to chest pain patients? I guess that's the end of that for us, huh?"

"Not really," Mary explained. "Using exploded search terms gets you a bunch of stuff that doesn't really fit. So, for example, some of those papers were about that new artificial blood stuff, diaspirin hemoglobin or something like that. Anyway, the search engine picks up the *aspirin* in *diaspirin* and adds that to the list. We had to go through the abstracts of the 29 articles and figure out which ones were really about aspirin and chest pain. There were only seven that really fit."

"OK, so seven studies have been done. I'm still not sure why we'd need to do another one."

"Tom, if you don't want to help, just say so, but don't be so negative." Mary was growing frustrated. She grabbed the pile of papers away from Tom and then placed one down in front of him. "Look at this. It's a study about whether or not paramedics can learn the indications and contraindications for aspirin. It has nothing to do with whether it works."

She placed another paper in front of him. "This one was a chart review to see how frequently the emergency department staff gave aspirin to chest pain patients. It's not EMS, and it doesn't say whether aspirin worked, either."

She waved the rest of the stack in front of his face.

"Seven studies, and not one of them looks at what we're interested in. They all just assume earlier is better—just like you said the other day."

"Oh, so now you're saying none of these papers are helpful. Sure glad you spent all that time in the library." Now Tom was picking on her. "That was sure a big help. How much did this cost you, anyway?"

"The copies were a nickel a page, so I guess I spent about five bucks altogether. And actually, it was helpful. These papers will help a lot in figuring out how to design our—or I guess maybe *MY*—study. Plus, I still have to look at the references in these papers and see if there's anything in there that might be useful. So far, the only things *I've* seen talk about giving aspirin for 30 days and how that makes outcome for MI patients better, but *I* need to look a little more to see if there's anything else that might help with *my* study."

"OK, OK, I'm sorry. I'm still with you." Tom knew he had to spend the next 12 hours caged in an ambulance with Mary. He sure didn't need to have her upset with him. "It's just hard for me to imagine that all of these ambulances are carrying aspirin for chest pain patients if nobody really knows that it helps."

Welcome to the world of EMS," Mary said sarcastically. "Where have you been for the last 17 years?"

Chapter 5
Defining the Question and Formulating a Hypothesis

Once a research topic has been chosen and a thorough literature search has been completed, the investigator can begin to formulate a specific research question. As might be expected, the extent to which the original research topic has already been refined and narrowed will influence, to a large extent, the amount of work required to craft a good research question. The information gleaned from the literature search will also influence the development of the question. What might be unexpected is that the work of defining the research question may cause the investigator to go back and rethink the topic, or to repeat and broaden the literature search. While research can be thought of as a step-by-step process, with each step affecting all future steps, it is in many ways a cyclical process. At each step along the way, at least during the early stages, the researcher may have to return to earlier steps and repeat or revise those pieces of the project. It is important to do this in the early stages because changes are not possible once the protocol is finalized and implemented. Defining the research question is likely to be the first point at which the researcher encounters this phenomenon. It will not be the last.

Knowing that future steps in the research process will probably cause the investigator to come back to and revise the question, it makes good sense to keep all of the future steps in mind when formulating the research question. If a researcher has decided to do a retrospective chart review to get a little experience before taking on a larger study, or to develop background information for a prospective study, it won't make sense to ask a question that can only be answered through a prospective, randomized controlled trial. If a researcher knows that the local institutional review board will not approve a waiver of consent in pediatric patients, it might not be a good idea to ask a question about pediatric cardiac arrest resuscitation. That's not to say that those wouldn't be good questions, just to say that an investigator must be realistic about what he or she can achieve.

DEVELOPING THE QUESTION

Based on the original research topic, the results of the literature search, and some understanding of what might happen in future steps, the investigator begins to define a research question. In the early stages of this process, it may be useful to simply brainstorm, writing down any and every question that comes to mind. Unlike the brainstorming for ideas conducted earlier, at this point all of the questions should relate to the chosen topic. Still, almost any question should be included at this point. Deciding which questions to drop and which to further refine can be done later. Also, don't worry about exact wording or grammatical issues at this point. Simply getting a laundry list of questions down on paper is an important first step. It gets the process started.

From the list of brainstormed questions, select two or three that seem to best address the research topic. Write them out, and begin to examine them to determine which—if any—of them asks the right question. It's amazing how often an investigator formulates a research question, only to find that the question doesn't really ask what he or she wanted to know. Be careful, and be nitpicky. This will be incredibly helpful when it comes time to narrow and refine the question.

It is also important at this point to make sure that the question is a question. Too often researchers establish an agenda, a point that they want to prove, and then try to disguise it as a question. Indeed, the process (as will be discussed in the section on hypothesis testing) should be the exact opposite: Choose a question, then suggest an answer to attempt to prove or disprove. It may seem like a purely academic differentiation, but in fact it will have a profound impact on the design, implementation, and eventual success of the research project.

Having identified one, two, or three questions that seem to best target the issue of interest, start trying to state each question in the form of a short, grammatically correct sentence. As with the process of identifying a topic, the idea is to repeatedly narrow and refine each question, getting it as specific as possible. Less is more. As the questions become more specific, review each one to determine that it is indeed a question and not a point to be proven; that it is a question that should be asked; and that it isn't going to cause conflicts at later points in the research process. Then, if more than one question meets those criteria, pick the one that inspires the most interest. Don't discard the other questions, though. As the process continues, the chosen question may not work out, and the investigator will need to return to these other options. Or, even if the chosen question does become the study question, the other questions may be appropriate options for future research projects.

REFINING THE QUESTION

At this point, the research question should be very focused. Yet, as the process continues, the researcher will find that the question will probably require even further refinement. Although it is a tedious process, developing a solid research question is critical to the success of any research project. The following is an example of how a brainstormed question relating to the topic of fluid resuscitation might be continuously refined into a narrow, focused question:

"Do intravenous fluids make a difference?"
"Do intravenous fluids make a difference for trauma patients?"

"Do intravenous fluids affect the outcome of trauma patients?"

"Do intravenous fluids affect survival in trauma patients?"

"Do intravenous fluids improve survival in trauma patients?"

"Do intravenous fluids improve survival in blunt trauma patients?"

"Do intravenous fluids improve survival to hospital admission in blunt trauma patients?"

At first blush, this appears to be a pretty good question and might make a good title for a paper, but as a question it still requires further refinement. What kind of fluids? What is "survival to hospital admission"? Is the question about all blunt trauma patients, or just those with chest and/or abdominal injuries? All of these points will have to be clarified in order to continue the research process.

To some extent, the researcher is now faced with a balancing act: making the question narrow and specific while keeping it short and clear. There's no absolute rule as to how to do this. It is not necessary to include each and every detail within the study question; all of those issues will be addressed in the design of the study. Still, the question must be as specific as possible and include measurable endpoints. One exercise that might help the researcher determine if the question is in fact well defined is to share the question with others who are not involved in the project and who are not aware of the investigator's specific interests or biases. Ask those people to read the question and to interpret it as they understand it. If everyone interprets the question exactly as the researcher intends, then the question is probably sufficient. If—as is more likely—the researcher hears several differing interpretations of the question, it needs more work.

After developing a question that is narrow and focused, that asks the right question, and that means the same thing to all who have reviewed it, the next step is to determine if it is a good question. Good, in this sense, doesn't mean well written or well formed, but practical and worthwhile. One approach to analyzing research questions that has been described by other researchers is to make sure it is a "FINER" research question. FINER stands for feasible, interesting, novel, ethical, and relevant. Examine the question. Is it *feasible?* Can it be done? Can it be done within the existing time and budget constraints? Can it be done within the existing system? Is it an *interesting* question? Will others be interested in and use the results? Is it *novel?* Is it a new area of research? Or, is it a new or better approach to an existing area of research? Is it *ethical?* Will the IRB approve the study? Could the results be used to bring harm—physical, emotional, economic, professional, or otherwise—to someone? Is it *relevant?* Will the results be applicable in the real world? Will the results be applicable in other systems? While it may be difficult for a researcher to objectively evaluate his or her own question, this is an important process and the successful researcher will learn to work through these issues without bias.

STATING THE QUESTION

Having decided upon a question, and having determined that the question is appropriate, the next step is to write it down in final form. While this seems like an obvious and easy step, it may not be. Look at each and every word. Is it really the right word? Will it have the same meaning to everyone? Does it reflect the researcher's bias? Yes, this is "wordsmithing," and while it's best to avoid such specificity in the early stages of defining the question, it must be done at this point. Hopefully, the earlier work of narrowing and refining the question will reduce the amount of rephrasing required at this point. Indeed, if the question requires a lot of revision at this point, it would probably be best to repeat the entire process. It can be a lot of work, with a lot of repetition and a lot of rehashing, but determining the research question is critical to the entire research process.

Some researchers use standard formats for their research questions. One common format that has been described and used extensively in the evidence-based medicine community is PICO. Unlike the FINER system discussed earlier, PICO applies to the specific question format, not the general suitability of the question. PICO questions identify the *patients* to be studied, the *interventions* to be performed, the *control* (or comparison) group(s) to be used, and the *outcomes* to be measured. Examining the final research question to determine how well it fits into the PICO model can help to ensure that the question is well written.

Now, after more work than most people would ever imagine, a final research question has emerged. What started as a broad area of interest has been repeatedly narrowed and refined, becoming more and more specific. As the question became more focused, it was reexamined to ensure that it was indeed a question and not a point to be proven. It was tested with peers to be certain that it was clear, and that everyone agreed on what the question asked. It was tested to be sure that it was an appropriate question, that it was doable, meaningful, and measurable. It was written out in final form, and once again evaluated to ensure that it had all of the components necessary for a good research question. But the process is not yet finished.

FORMULATING THE HYPOTHESIS

Now the question must be formed into a hypothesis—a statement of fact that the study will attempt to prove or disprove. Often, a well-crafted question can easily be transformed into a hypothesis simply by rearranging the words. For example, the question, "Does restricting fluid administration improve survival to hospital discharge in children with blunt head injuries?" could be restated as the hypothesis, "Restricting fluid administration improves survival to hospital discharge in children with blunt head injuries." Or, the question, "Do commercial head immobilizers provide better cervical stabilization than towel rolls and tape in the immobilized adult?" could be restated as the hypothesis, "Commercial head immobilizers provide better cervical stabilization than towel rolls and tape in the immobilized adult."

For more complex or broader questions, it may be more difficult to formulate a hypothesis. Some questions may include more than one hypothesis. Generally, questions that generate more than one hypothesis might best be answered in two or more different studies, but there are times when a single study can address two hypotheses. For example, a question such as, "Is paramedic student success related to previous health care experience or years of EMS experience?" is really two questions: "Is paramedic student success related to previous health care experience?" and "Is paramedic student success related to years of EMS experience?" In a retrospective review of student records, it might make as much sense to explore these two issues simultaneously as separately. Still, each poses its own hypothesis: "Paramedic student success is related to previous health care experience" and "Paramedic student success is related to years of EMS experience." While data collection for these two hypotheses may be simultaneous, each should be evaluated independently.

It might be tempting at this point to add a third question and its subsequent hypothesis, "Years of EMS experience are more important than previous health care experience in paramedic student success." Be careful! That is a distinct question, a new hypothesis, and probably the beginnings of a different study. It wouldn't be a bad study, and the researcher may want to go back to the topic and the literature search and explore whether or not its actually a better question, or at least a question that better addresses the interests of the researcher. The investigator should not, however, add more and more questions—and more and more hypotheses—to the study. If there appear to be several hypotheses suggested by the research question, it generally means that the research question is not well defined. The investigator should return to the beginning of the process and refine the topic and the question.

This process of refinement, revision, and reevaluation repeating over and over does seem troublesome, and it can slow the research process. It is, however, extremely important. An unclear question produces a nonspecific hypothesis, which usually results in a useless study. A recent study by an EMS graduate student provides a good example of this. The topic was good: wellness among EMS providers. The question—is wellness related to longevity in EMS?—was not as good. The hypothesis was never truly developed, and the method for measuring wellness was never defined. A survey with about 70 questions was mailed to hundreds of EMS providers, and the responses generated thousands of data points. Unfortunately, since there was no predetermined hypothesis, there wasn't any good way to analyze the data. Comparing the relationships among each of the 70 or so variables with each of the other 70 or so variables would produce just under 2500 two-by-two tables. While that's a lot of data, there's no reasonable way to interpret it. Had the study specifically hypothesized a relationship between diet and longevity, or spirituality and longevity, or a specific validated wellness score and longevity, the data would have been much more useful.

The hypothesis should be a single declarative sentence. Usually, a hypothesis is short and to the point. In general, hypotheses should not include conjunctions such as *and, or,* and *but* or words and phrases like *because, in order to, instead of,* or *in addition to.* These phrases suggest that the study is exploring more than one issue. For example, the study question, "Do volunteer paramedics have poorer intubation success rates than urban paramedics because they have lower call volumes?" actually involves two issues: "Do volunteer paramedics have lower intubation success rates than urban paramedics?" and "Is intubation success related to call volume?" Thus, there are two distinct hypotheses to be tested: "Volunteer paramedics have lower intubation success rates than urban paramedics" and "Intubation success rates are affected by call volume." Is that nitpicky? Yes, but confusing the two issues could absolutely have an adverse effect on the entire research process.

There are a few cases in which a hypothesis will not have to be developed. Descriptive studies that simply explore the current status of any given topic or a specific population may not require a specific hypothesis. Such studies, though, are inherently weak and can rarely be used to answer questions or formulate policy. Describing the previous health care experience of successful paramedic students is not the same as testing the hypothesis that there is a relationship between previous experience and success.

THE NULL HYPOTHESIS

There is one last step in developing the question and the hypothesis, and that is to formulate the null hypothesis. The null hypothesis is the opposite of what one expects to find, and can usually be crafted rather simply from the hypothesis.

Consider the question, "Does restricting administration of intravenous crystalloids improve survival to hospital discharge in patients with blunt head injuries?" The hypothesis would be, "Restricting administration of intravenous crystalloids improves survival to hospital discharge in patients with blunt head injuries." The null hypothesis would be, "Restricting administration of intravenous crystalloids *does not* improve survival to hospital discharge in patients with blunt head injuries."

Yes, this is more wordsmithing, and some researchers omit this step in the research process. The development of the null hypothesis is crucial to the research process, however. While it may seem like an academic endeavor, testing the null hypothesis is the basis for all true research.

HYPOTHESIS TESTING

The reasons for developing a null hypothesis are based in logic. The null hypothesis is a "straw man" that the investigator attempts to knock down through the research process. If the null hypothesis can be disproved or rejected, then the alternative—the hypothesis—can be accepted. While this seems convoluted, it is the essence of scientific analysis and will affect all aspects of any proposed study. Designing a study that attempts to reject a null hypothesis is very different than designing a study that attempts to prove a hypothesis. Testing a null hypothesis is one of the most effective ways to avoid bias and error in a study. There are other ways, but this approach is one of the most basic tenets of the research process.

Think about it in practical terms. If someone has proposed a new method of airway management and is trying to convince the EMS community that it is a better approach, that person can take two different approaches. That person could design a study that attempts to prove that his or her idea is better (i.e., that attempts to prove the hypothesis). Or, that person could design a study that attempts to prove that his or her idea is not better (i.e., that attempts to prove the null hypothesis).

In testing the hypothesis, "My idea is better," the study methodology would be developed to prove "my idea is better" and the analysis would be geared toward proving "my idea is better." Thus, it wouldn't be much of a surprise when the study results in fact suggested that "my idea *is* better." Most people, however, would be skeptical of the conclusions, and worry that the investigator's bias affected everything from the initial conceptualization of the study all the way through the final data analysis and interpretation.

If, on the other hand, the investigator attempts to prove the null hypothesis, "My idea is not better," then the study design would be developed to prove "my idea is not better" and the data analysis would be geared toward proving "my idea is not better." If the study fails to prove "my idea is not better," then that statement is rejected. Logically then, the remaining option—the alternative hypothesis that "my idea is better"—can be accepted. As long as people are able to review the study design and assure themselves that the approach was valid and the attempt to prove the null hypothesis was sincere, they can have confidence in the results of the study and in the acceptance of the alternative hypothesis.

In the crystalloid study example, the researchers would attempt to prove that there is no difference in the survival rates of patients who have fluids restricted and those who do not. Some patients would have their fluids restricted and others would not. At the end of the study, survival to hospital discharge for the two groups would be compared. If the survival rate in the group with restricted fluids was greater than that in the other group (if the researchers were unable to prove that there is no difference), then the null hypothesis would be rejected. The alternative—the hypothesis that restricting fluid does improve outcome—would then be logically accepted.

It might be tempting for a researcher to develop a hypothesis and a methodology for testing that hypothesis, and then to formulate a null hypothesis for the sake of the abstract or the manuscript. That misses the point completely, and will become obvious when readers examine the study methodology. Developing and testing a null hypothesis is the appropriate way to reach research conclusions. While it may be confusing to think about, it is no more difficult than trying to prove a hypothesis. The important thing is that the results of testing a null hypothesis are always more meaningful.

SUMMARY

Developing the research question and hypothesis, like all of the steps in the research process, is built upon the previous steps and will influence all future steps. Also, like all other components of the research process, the act of developing the question might cause the investigator to go back and revisit previous steps and future steps might cause the researcher to come back and revisit the question. The whole process is cyclical.

The question is built out of the study topic, and simple brainstorming is the easiest way to begin to formulate questions. From the brainstormed list of questions, a researcher can choose the one or two that best address the issue at hand and begin to refine those questions. The process is designed to make the question as specific and narrow as possible.

Once the question has been formulated and refined, the researcher can develop a hypothesis. The hypothesis should be a single statement of fact representing what the researcher expects to find as a result of the study. From the hypothesis, the researcher can create the null hypothesis, which will become the basis for the study design. The study will attempt to prove the null hypothesis. If it is unable to do so, the null hypothesis can be rejected and the alternative—the original hypothesis—can be accepted.

While the repetitiveness required in refining the question and the hypothesis can be frustrating, taking time to work through the process at this early stage will pay off in the long run. Good questions and good hypotheses lead to good studies.

A Typical Experience
Part 3: Defining the Question and Formulating a Hypothesis

It had been about two weeks since Mary and Tom had first cooked up their research idea. They still talked about it on every shift, but the level of enthusiasm had been waning for both of them. Mary had been trying to read all of the journal articles she had found. Getting through the original seven articles hadn't taken too long, but she now had another half dozen articles identified from the references of those papers.

"I keep finding more and more stuff, and it's all pretty interesting, but none of these studies really answers my—er, I mean *our*—question."

"Yeah," Tom said, "but now you know more about aspirin and chest pain than anyone else working in this system. They should have you teach a continuing education class or something."

"Right. On how not to try to start a research project."

"Aw, c'mon, Mary." Tom could see she was getting discouraged. "I think you're farther along than you think. You know, this isn't something you can just cook up overnight and finish in a few days."

"I know," Mary continued in a tired voice, "but I'm not even sure I know what my—I mean *our*—research question is."

"I thought it was whether or not aspirin made a difference for chest pain patients."

"Well, yeah, but it really needs to be more specific than that, Tom. I've been talking with my neighbor who teaches statistics at the community college, and she says one thing to be really careful about is to have a very specific, very focused research question."

"What's more focused than chest pain and aspirin?" Tom asked.

"I've been thinking about that a lot. After reading all of these papers, I've got a better idea about how those seemingly simple words and phrases can mean entirely different things. Like, when we say *chest pain,* do we mean patients with any chest pain? Or only patients having angina? Or, do we really mean patients who are having an MI? When we say *makes a difference,* do we mean whether or not the patient dies? Or do we mean whether or not they get thrombolytics? Do we mean how big their infarct is? Or do we mean how many days they spend in the ICU?"

"Jeez, Mary, you're sure making this complicated!"

"Yeah, well, this isn't something you can just cook up overnight," she grinned.

"Touché!" Tom laughed. "I'll tell you what. After our shift let's go grab a burger and spend a little time figuring out exactly what it is we want to get at."

The rest of the shift was largely uneventful. They responded to one car crash in a nearby parking lot where nobody was really hurt, even though one of the drivers wanted to go to the hospital to get checked out. They also had an elderly man with respiratory distress who seemed to be doing pretty well after a couple of breathing treatments. In between they had two convalescent transports from one of the nursing homes to a doctor's office, and then back again.

Now, they looked down at the legal pad in the middle of the orange linoleum tabletop. They had been brainstorming for about 15 minutes. Tom brushed aside a loose french fry that had fallen from his tray and was leaving a greasy stain on the yellow paper. "That's quite a list," he said.

They had nearly filled the legal pad with questions—one written on every other line:

Is aspirin helpful for chest pain patients?

Is prehospital administration of aspirin helpful for chest pain patients?

How many chest pain patients really have an MI?

Is prehospital aspirin helpful for patients having an MI?

Does prehospital aspirin administration reduce mortality in MI?

Does prehospital aspirin administration reduce mortality in angina?

Does EMS aspirin administration speed delivery of thrombolytics in the ED?

Is giving aspirin more important than starting an IV for chest pain patients?

Does nitroglycerin reduce mortality in angina patients?

Does nitroglycerin reduce the rate of MI in chest pain patients?

Is giving nitroglycerin more important that giving aspirin in chest pain patients?

Is survival of MI patients higher in EMS systems that give aspirin than in systems that don't?

What is the best measure of whether something "helps" for chest pain patients?

Is giving aspirin in the field better than giving aspirin in the emergency department for chest pain patients?

Do chest pain patients who get their aspirin in the field do better than those who get their aspirin in the emergency room?

Do cardiac patients who get prehospital aspirin have better outcomes than those who get aspirin in the emergency department?

Mary read over the list again. "You know, I don't think we're quite there yet, but this really is helping me think through things. What do you think of this?" She took the pad, tore off the top sheet, and on the next one wrote:

In EMS patients with suspected cardiac chest pain, does administering aspirin in the prehospital setting result in lower mortality when compared to waiting to administer the aspirin at the hospital?

"I thought it was supposed to be simple and focused," Tom said. "That seems like a pretty long-winded question."

"Yeah, it's not perfect, but it's getting closer. I know it's been a long day, but what do you say we go over to the main station and see what the folks there think about it?"

"Works for me," Tom said as he stood up and began to clear away the hamburger wrappers and paper cups. "I have no life—I might as well hang with you for a while."

Timmy had been a paramedic for about 12 years, and had actually participated in a couple of studies that some of the local physicians had done. "So, you want to know if giving aspirin to cardiac patients in the field reduces the death rate, instead of giving it in the ED," he said as he passed the legal pad back to Tom.

"Exactly," Mary smiled. She turned to Tom, "All the other people knew what we were trying to get at too, so maybe our question isn't so bad after all."

"Hold on there." Timmy rocked back in his chair with his arms folded across his chest. He had a smug look on his face that—for a moment, anyway—made Mary hope that he'd topple over backwards. "Just because I knew what you meant doesn't mean it's a good question. I don't think there's any way you can do this study."

Tom barked, "Well, pal, that's why nobody here pays you to think." He didn't like Timmy. "We're not even close to figuring out how to do this yet, we're just trying to make sure that we've got a question that means the same thing to everyone. Even you."

Mary was astounded. She never expected to see Tom actively defending the research project. She figured he had just been patronizing her because they were partners. "Calm down, Tom. We do still have to make sure that this study is doable. Not all good questions can be studied, and we do have to think about that."

"Yeah, you're right. *We* need to think about that."

"I found this little guide," Mary said as she searched through her bookbag. "It says one way to evaluate a research question is to use this FINER technique. It stands for . . ." she hesitated as she searched for the booklet. "Oh, here it is." She flipped through the pages. "Feasible, interesting, novel, ethical, and relevant."

"Well," Tom spoke proudly, with a cutting glance at Timmy, "we know it's novel since nobody else has done it yet. And it's certainly relevant. We're giving aspirin to every chest pain patient."

"It's interesting to us," Mary continued, "and I can't imagine why it would be unethical to study this."

"But it's that feasible piece that's going to give you trouble," Timmy interjected, now leaning even further back and looking so smug that Mary thought—now for more than just a moment—about reaching out and pushing him over.

"Well, that's for us to figure out. Come on, Tom. Let's go see if we can turn this into a grammatically correct sentence so we can formulate a hypothesis. I think we're pretty close."

It took about another hour, but when Mary and Tom were done, they not only had a clear question; they had even applied another guideline—PICO—to make sure that it specifically identified the patients, the intervention, the comparison group, and the outcome of interest.

Mary read aloud: "Do EMS patients treated under the cardiac chest pain protocol who receive aspirin in the prehospital setting have lower mortality rates than those in whom aspirin administration is delayed until arrival at the emergency department?"

"So that makes the hypothesis," Tom added. "EMS patients treated under the cardiac chest pain protocol who receive aspirin in the prehospital setting have lower mortality rates than those in whom aspirin administration is delayed until arrival at the emergency department."

"And the null hypothesis . . ."

They spoke in unison, "EMS patients treated under the cardiac chest pain protocol who receive aspirin in the prehospital setting *do not* have lower mortality rates than those in whom aspirin administration is delayed until arrival at the emergency department."

"We did it!"

"Yeah," Tom said. "Now we just need to figure out how to really do the study, or we're going to have to listen to Timmy gloat for the rest of our careers."

"Ha!" laughed Mary. "What better motivation could there be?"

SECTION 3

DESIGNING THE STUDY

Chapter 6

Determining the
Type of Study

Once the researcher has developed a question and formulated a hypothesis, the next step is to decide upon the type of study to be conducted. In addition to determining whether the study will be retrospective or prospective and whether it will be quantitative or qualitative, the investigator must decide how the study subjects will be identified and how the study factor—if there is one—will be allocated. These decisions will greatly affect the study methodology, and the process of determining the type of study and developing the methodology may take place simultaneously. The two processes, though, are distinct, and this chapter focuses on determining the type of study.

LOW-TECH STUDIES

Descriptive Studies

Probably the lowest-tech, least scientific methodology for a study is a descriptive study. Descriptive studies are, by their nature, observational studies. They can be qualitative or quantitative, and they can be prospective or retrospective. There is no control group; there is no randomization.

In a descriptive study, there really isn't a study factor or intervention. No hypothesis is tested. The researcher collects information about the way something is (or was) in one or more EMS systems. Typically the study is done to collect data that will allow the researcher to describe an event, an approach, or perhaps a unique piece of equipment. A descriptive study could describe the approach a system took to address a specific problem. A descriptive study could describe the patient care protocols different systems have for certain chief complaints. A descriptive study could explain how an entire EMS system developed.

Some EMS researchers—indeed, some researchers in general—trivialize the value of descriptive studies. However, EMS is a relatively young component of the medical community, and there is still great variability from system to system. Learning from the experiences of others is important. Certainly, broad-reaching policy decisions should be based on more sophisticated science, but knowing what other people and other systems are doing is valuable. There is no reason to reinvent the wheel; there is no reason to repeat someone else's failures. While descriptive studies do not answer specific questions or test hypotheses, they do have value in developing a basic understanding of EMS practices.

Quality Improvement Studies

Perhaps the easiest and most common approach to EMS research is to use data from a system's existing quality improvement program. Usually such projects are retrospective, observational studies, and sometimes they are purely descriptive. But it is possible to conduct a quality improvement study that does have a study factor. It is even possible to conduct a prospective, maybe even quasi-experimental, quality improvement study.

If the researcher describes intubation success rates over the past 3 years, that is a retrospective descriptive study. If the researcher decides today that he or she is going to collect intubation data for the next 6 months, that will make the project prospective. If the researcher looks at intubation success rates before and after changing to disposable laryngoscopes—either retrospectively or prospectively—that will make it a quasi-experimental study.

One shortcoming of quality assurance–type research is that the data are really collected for another reason. That makes it hard to collect all of the data needed without having to sort through a bunch of other data that the QI people want but the researcher doesn't. Another shortcoming is that most EMS providers are usually aware when something is being targeted in the QI program, and they may make some extra effort to do that thing—whatever it is—well. This is known as the Hawthorne effect: When people know they're being watched, they behave differently.

Still, especially for the new researcher, existing QI programs can be a great source for data. The new researcher has to start somewhere, and there's nothing wrong with making things a little easier for the first few studies. Like descriptive studies, QI studies from one system may help others figure out what to do in their systems. They can lead to bigger and better questions, and sometimes can even be a catalyst for change within an EMS system.

Surveys and Questionnaires

On the surface, a survey or questionnaire may appear to be an easy way to approach a research question. Surveys are prospective, and they can be observational, quasi-experimental, or experimental.

A one-time survey of EMTs about the type of ambulance they prefer would be observational. If a researcher surveys a group of EMTs that all use type II ambulances now, and then surveys them again 6 months after they switch to type III ambulances, that is quasi-experimental. If a researcher surveys a group of EMTs now, then randomizes them to receive an advertisement promoting one or the other type of ambulance, and then surveys them again, that is experimental.

The problem with surveys is that it's almost impossible to get them to ask exactly what the researcher wants to ask. If fill-in-the-blank responses are used, the data become qualitative—and almost impossible to analyze. If strict multiple-choice responses are used, some participants may not like the choices they're given. They may leave spaces blank—or worse, make up and write in their own choices!

Another difficult thing is making sure the participants understand the question the way it's intended. Imagine the many different ways someone could answer the question: "How many of your patients are ugly?" In a week? In a year? Should the answer be a number or a percentage? The problem is, just because the researcher knows what he or she intends to ask, that doesn't mean the respondent will know. And, if the respondent *does* know exactly what's being asked—and thinks he or she knows exactly what the researcher wants to hear—the response may be what the respondent thinks the researcher is looking for, not the truth. It's the Hawthorne effect again. The subjects know they're being watched, so they may respond differently than they would otherwise. A final problem with surveys can be recall bias. People don't always remember things exactly as they happened, especially if the survey asks about things that happened some time ago.

Surveys can be effective, and they require relatively few resources, but they demand a more refined level of expertise than most people think. Good researchers who undertake surveys always find someone with experience in the area to help design the survey, and they always do a pilot test. Still, if a researcher is really interested in what people think, then a survey may be an appropriate approach.

MID-TECH STUDIES

Case Control Studies

In a case control study, the researcher identifies two groups of people: one with a specific disease or outcome, one without. Then all of the other characteristics of the two groups are evaluated to determine if one or more of those characteristics could explain why the disease developed in one group and not the other. Case control studies are observational studies: The researcher does not control any study factor. In fact, the researcher is trying to figure out what are the factors that affect the outcome.

A real-life example of this occurred in the 1980s, when there was a large incidence of Reye's syndrome. Doctors identified two groups of children: those with flulike symptoms who developed Reye's, and those with flulike symptoms who did not. They then searched through the medical histories of all the patients and found that the children who developed Reye's were more likely to have been given aspirin than were those who did not. While that study did not prove beyond all doubt that aspirin causes Reye's, it did demonstrate a significant association between the two, and it radically changed aspirin administration practices.

An example of an EMS case control study could be to examine patients with penetrating trauma. A researcher could identify two groups of patients who were shot through the heart: one group of survivors and one group of nonsurvivors. Then the researcher would search through the histories of both groups of patients to see if there were anything that could explain why some died and some lived. Of course, there would be hundreds of things to examine: response time, scene time, intravenous fluids, oxygen flow rates, distance to the hospital, whether the patients went to a trauma center, and so on. The researcher must pick the one or two things that are most likely to explain the difference, and incorporate those into the hypothesis. It is possible that the researcher will find that these things don't explain the difference, leaving open the question of what other things might be responsible. That can be one of the problems with case control studies—it can be like looking for a needle in a haystack, without knowing for sure that there's really a needle in there.

The greatest difficulty in a case control study is making sure that the controls (the group without the disease or outcome) are otherwise very similar to the cases (those with the disease or outcome). If all the victims of penetrating trauma who lived were under 30 years of age and all those who died were over 30, the difference in survival may be due to the difference in age, not to anything that happened in the patients' prehospital care. If all those who died were shot with high-powered rifles and all those who lived were shot with handguns, that alone might explain the difference. Differences in prehospital care might not be the culprit at all.

Historical Prospective Studies

Historical prospective studies are a little different from case control studies. Historical prospective studies are observational, too. There is a study factor of interest, but the researcher does not control it. Sometimes these are called retrospective cohort studies, and sometimes they are called before-and-after studies.

In a historical prospective study, the researcher selects a single group of subjects, independent of whatever disease or outcome they may have. Then the researcher looks into the past records of those people (or just asks them) to determine if they had an exposure to the study factor of interest. From that baseline, the researcher then determines who ended up with the disease or outcome of interest.

Suppose an EMS researcher is trying to determine whether EMTs trained by male instructors are more likely to have heart attacks than those trained by female instructors. First a group of EMTs has to be selected: perhaps all of the students trained in one state during the past 5 years. Then the researcher determines their exposure to the study factor by determining whether their very first EMT instructor was a man or a woman. The EMTs can then be divided into two groups based on the sex of their first instructor: a group of EMTs trained by women, and a group trained by men. Now, all that has to be done is to track these EMTs for the next 5 years to see who does and who doesn't have a heart attack. In the end, the researcher can compare the proportion of EMTs trained by women who have heart attacks to the proportion of EMTs trained by men who have heart attacks. Who trained them is historical; it constitutes retrospective data. Whether or not the EMT has a heart attack is prospective.

An obvious limitation to an historical prospective approach is that the prospective part has to have an endpoint. There's no way to know what might happen after the 5-year study is over. Twenty years later the heart attack data might look very different.

HI-TECH STUDIES

Cross-Sectional Studies

Cross-sectional studies are a snapshot of a population at a specific time. Actually, some of the low- and mid-tech designs can also be considered cross-sectional. A survey, for example, is a snapshot of those who respond. A quality assurance study is a snapshot of that system at that point in time.

Cross-sectional studies are a reasonable way to measure associations between two or more things, and they can be considerably more sophisticated than a survey. Chan's study about vacuum splints and traditional backboards was a cross-sectional study.[3] It used 37 volunteers—a cross section of the population—and examined them over a little more than 2 weeks—a cross section of time. The strength of a cross-sectional study is in picking a sample that is a reliable cross section of the real world. If the 37 volunteers were all patients with arthritis, for example, they wouldn't be a realistic cross section. If, on the other hand, they were all people with a driver's license who had been involved in at least one motor vehicle collision, then they would be a reasonable cross section of people likely to be immobilized.

Cohort Studies

Cohort studies are prospective studies that compare two or more groups of patients to see what effect different study factors have on their outcomes. The allocation of the study factor is used to sort the people into groups, and then they are followed to see what outcome develops.

One example of a cohort study is the MAST study that was conducted in Houston, Texas.[4] That was a quasi-experimental study where some trauma patients with low blood pressure got MAST (the MAST cohort), and others did not get MAST (the no-MAST cohort). The design was quasi-experimental because the MAST and no-MAST allocations were alternated, not randomized. The patients were followed to see if their outcomes were different. That study demonstrated that MAST increased mortality for patients with penetrating chest trauma.

Randomized Controlled Trials

The highest-tech research is the randomized controlled trial (RCT). RCTs are prospective, experimental cohort studies. In these studies, the study factor is allocated in a completely randomized fashion; the researcher has no control over how it is distributed. The participants are followed to see if they develop different outcomes. The most sophisticated form of a randomized controlled trial is the double-blind study. Double-blind means that neither the researcher nor the patient knows which intervention is allocated to that subject. This is important because of the Hawthorne effect. If patients know whether or not they received real medicine or a placebo, their outcome might be affected by what they think the outcome should be. And researchers, no matter how hard they try, can't be totally objective, either. So if the researcher knows whether the patient received an active medication or placebo, he or she might look harder for the outcome, or wait just a little longer to collect the data, or potentially bias the study in some other way. In the best studies, neither the patient nor the researcher knows whether the subject was in the control or the intervention group.

Perhaps one of the best examples of an EMS double-blind randomized controlled trial was conducted by Zehner et al.[5] This was a study to determine if asthma patients experienced better relief of symptoms when they were treated with subcutaneous terbutaline or nebulized albuterol. The EMS providers enrolled all of the asthma patients they encountered. The pharmacy put together blinded packages of medication so that neither the paramedics, the researchers, nor the patients knew what medication any patient got. To do this, the patient had to get both a subcutaneous injection and a breathing treatment. One of these (but only the pharmacist knew which) was just saline, and one was real medicine. The medication packets were coded, and the paramedics recorded the code, gave the patient the medicines, and then recorded whether or not the patient got better. The doctors in the emergency department recorded whether or not the patient needed more treatments, and what the patient's final outcome was. The pharmacist didn't break the code for the study packets until all of the patients had been enrolled and all of the important information had been recorded. Only then could the researcher analyze the data and determine that albuterol provided greater relief of symptoms than did terbutaline.

DETERMINING THE TYPE OF STUDY

The type of study chosen depends on many factors, including the question to be answered, the resources available, and the expertise of the researcher. A descriptive approach would not be appropriate for testing a hypothesis. A survey wouldn't be the best way to determine the differences in the effects of two medications. A randomized controlled trial might be too great an undertaking for a new researcher.

While higher-tech studies might be more rigorous and provide stronger answers, they require more resources and greater expertise. Lower-tech studies are easier to implement and require fewer resources, but they are less scientific. There is no right answer when determining the type of study to be performed. The investigator has to balance all of the issues associated with study design and choose the approach with the greatest chance for success.

SUMMARY

Once the study hypothesis is formulated, the researcher has to determine the type of study that will be conducted. The study type will greatly influence the study methodology. There are many types of studies; some are more scientific than others. The researcher must balance the desire for a rigorous design with the realities of available resources and the investigator's expertise. No single type of study is truly the best; the investigator has to choose the approach that is most likely to lead to a successful project.

A Typical Experience
Part 4: Determining the Type of Study

"So Tom, how are we going to do this study? Timmy was harassing me the other day, and I really don't want him to be right about this."

Tom looked across the stretcher at Mary. "You think I do? I've actually been surfing around the Internet looking for information on doing clinical studies. I can't believe I'm actually spending my own time working on this! You're turning me into one of those research geeks."

"See, that's a good thing." Checking to be sure that the stretcher was secured, Mary closed the two rear doors to the ambulance and sat down on the bumper. "You've always been a geek, Tom. Now you can be a specialist."

"Whatever. Anyway, it seems like all the easy ways to do a study wouldn't really answer our question. The types of studies that would probably get us a good answer all seem hard to do. We may have bitten off more than we can chew."

Dave Walsh, one of the ED doctors, tapped on the side of the ambulance as he came around to the back. "What did you two bring us?"

"Oh, hey, doc." Mary stood up to shake his hand. Tom just nodded. "Another chest pain patient. We gave him some aspirin and saved his life."

"You're starting to sound as cynical as Tom, Mary." Dave jabbed Tom in the belly with his index finger. "We might have to split you two up."

"Promise?" Tom smiled, pushing Dave's hand away.

"Hey!" Mary protested. "Actually, neither one of us is really that cynical about this. We've just been talking a lot lately about whether or not giving aspirin in the field really makes a difference."

"Well," Dave offered, "a true cynic might wonder whether anything you guys do makes any difference."

"Thank you for your support," Mary said mockingly. "We're serious. We've been trying to figure out a way to study it. You got any bright ideas?"

"Hmmm. I guess the easy way would be to look at chest pain patients from back before you started giving aspirin, and compare them to the patients you've been bringing in ever since aspirin was added to the protocol. You could do that retrospectively, so it could be done pretty quickly."

"Problem," Tom said. "The ED started giving thrombolytics to MI patients about the same time we started giving aspirin, so any differences in their outcome might be because of that."

"What if we only looked at patients that didn't get thrombolytics?" Mary asked.

"No, I guess Tom is right, Mary. Since one of the reasons we withhold thrombolytics is when it's been too long since the chest pain started, that would mean a lot of the patients in your aspirin group would be patients who had been having pain for several hours. They might be predisposed to having worse outcomes."

Tom looked at the ground and shuffled his feet. "We could look back through the records for the last 3 years and pick out all of those patients I forgot to give aspirin to, and compare them to patients who were taken care of by good paramedics. I think the QI officer has a whole folder full of 'Tom's screwups.' They shouldn't be that hard to find."

Dave chuckled. "You'd have a hard time getting enough patients that way. You don't mess up *that much,* Tom."

"Gee, thanks, doc."

"Well, I've got to get to work, but I'm sure you two will figure something out. Let me know what I can do to help." Dave turned away and started through the sliding doors of the ambulance entrance.

"We will," Mary said. "I'm sure we'll need your approval for whatever we come up with. You are the medical director, after all."

"I am cursed, aren't I?" he shouted back over his shoulder, laughing.

"You know, Mary, there's no way we're going to be able to do this retrospectively," Tom said.

"Probably not," she conceded. "You realize it's going to take us a long time to do it prospectively, don't you?"

Tom playfully shook his finger at her. "I'm retiring in 8 years, whether this study is done or not!"

"Sure, old man. So, do we want to do something quasi-experimental, or do we want to go whole hog with a double-blind randomized trial?"

"I don't know. Which one will upset Timmy the most?"

Mary gave Tom a thumbs-up. "It scares me when we think so much alike. Do you really think we can pull off a randomized controlled study?"

"I think we should give it our best shot. Everything I've been reading says RCTs are the best way to investigate therapies, and aspirin *is* a therapy."

"An RCT it is then." Mary threw Tom the keys to the ambulance. "Right now we better get back in service. You're driving."

Chapter 7
Developing the Methods

When it comes to research, the devil *is* in the details.

Once the researcher has determined whether the study will be prospective or retrospective, and whether the design will be observational, quasi-experimental, or experimental, he or she must determine precisely how the study will be conducted. The methodology must be designed in a way that enables the study to answer the research question by proving or rejecting the study's null hypothesis. At the same time, the methodology must be realistic and feasible. Most importantly, the methodology must be detailed enough to ensure that everyone involved in the study knows exactly what to do, when to do it, and how to react to unforeseen circumstances.

Everything the investigator has done up to this point will influence the study methodology. For example, the original research topic will dictate where the study is conducted, and on what types of patients. The literature search will have provided information about methodologies used in similar studies, and what worked and what did not. The hypothesis will dictate what data are collected, and the study type will determine how those data are obtained. Indeed, as with every step in the research process, the investigator will likely revisit each of these previous steps while developing the study methodology.

IDENTIFYING THE POPULATION TO BE STUDIED

One piece of the methodology that may seem easy to define is the study population. In fact, defining the population is extremely important, and is often more difficult than one might imagine. At first, the investigator may simply identify the subjects based on the research topic. If the study is a clinical study, the subjects will be patients. If the project is an educational study, the subjects might be students or teachers. If the study involves systems research, the subjects might be entire EMS systems, administrators, or maybe—once again—patients.

The investigator undertaking a clinical study must carefully define the patients who will be included. If the study involves an approach to patient assessment, it might be feasible to include all of the patients transported by the system. If the study involves an intervention for asthma, it's probably not reasonable to include all patients. Should the study of an asthma intervention include all patients in respiratory distress, only those believed by paramedics to be having an asthma attack, or only those who are ultimately diagnosed by the emergency physician to be having an asthma attack? That decision must be made within the context of the research hypothesis: which group of patients will allow the researcher to best answer the question?

Once the researcher undertaking a clinical study has identified the appropriate group of subjects, those patients must still be better defined. There are other criteria that will influence whether a patient qualifies for enrollment in the study. For example, should age be a criterion? If the intervention were indicated only in adult patients, then clearly it would be inappropriate to include children. Now the researcher must decide the age at which patients would qualify for enrollment. The American Heart Association guidelines for cardiopulmonary resuscitation recommend "adult" interventions for anyone over 8 years of age. Children may mature physiologically at around 15 or 16 years of age. The IRB (which will require special consent procedures for children) will likely define children as patients under the age of 18 years. Finally, some children may be covered by their parents' health insurance up to the age of 25 years. Any one of these ages may be an appropriate cutoff for any given study. It's up to the researcher to consider all of these issues—and many others—and determine where the line will be drawn. There is no easy answer; it will be different for every study.

There are hundreds, if not thousands, of possible criteria to consider when defining the study population, but not all of them will apply to every study. It might be necessary to use physiologic parameters to identify patients, such as a respiratory rate of at least 26 or an altered level of consciousness. It might be appropriate to limit participants to those older than 50 years of age or to only those trauma victims who were ejected from their vehicles. Again, the idea is to select the best study population for addressing the research hypothesis.

The researcher must also consider and decide upon the exclusion criteria for the subjects. These are items that would make an otherwise eligible patient ineligible. An asthma study enrolling patients complaining of shortness of breath who are over the age of 50 and who have home nebulizers might want to exclude patients with certain co-morbid conditions, such as lung cancer. In a study enrolling ejected car crash victims to determine if the shape of the driver's side window contributes to the injury pattern, the investigator might want to exclude those patients ejected from a convertible with the top down. Part of the idea is to exclude those subjects whose condition or outcome might be influenced by things that are totally unrelated to the study, but another reason for exclusion criteria is to protect the subjects. In a study of fluid resuscitation in trauma patients, for example, the researcher would want to exclude patients with isolated head injuries, in whom fluid overload would be dangerous.

Identifying the study participants for an educational study can be just as complicated as identifying patients for a clinical study. All EMS courses, all EMS teachers, and all EMS students are not alike. Some EMS courses are taught as adult continuing education classes; some are taught as community college or university classes. Some EMS instructors are primarily clinicians whose careers have evolved so that they are now educators; some have formal training in education. Some EMS students are fresh out of high school with no medical background; some have been involved in EMS for dozens of years and are in the process of advancing their level of certification. It's not necessary for the researcher to make value judgements about these things, only to recognize and consider these issues when identifying the study population.

The inclusion criteria for an educational study will likely have to define at least three characteristics of the study subjects: Who are they, who is teaching them, and in what environment? The exclusion criteria must be defined, too. Should the study exclude students with other health care experience? Someone who is already an emergency department nurse is not a typical paramedic student. Should the study exclude people with certain formal education? Someone with a PhD in education will likely have better test-taking skills than a 22-year-old ex-marine who worked as a medic during her service years. As always, it's up to the investigator to identify these issues and to decide which ones should be used as inclusion and exclusion criteria, and which ones can be ignored.

Studies of EMS systems can be the most difficult for which to define the study population. If the research involves comparing systems, then those organizations need to be described in detail. As with clinical and education research, the inclusion and exclusion criteria will depend largely on what is being studied. If the research is testing the accuracy of a new computerized data collection program, differences between rural and urban systems may not be that important. On the other hand, if a study is examining the impact of the use of lights and sirens on response times, the differences between urban and rural systems might be quite important. For another perspective, consider a study that compares EMS agencies that employ system status management with those that respond from fixed stations. Who or what are the study subjects? If costs are being studied, then perhaps the systems and their respective budgets are the study subjects. If employee turnover is being studied, then perhaps the subjects are the individual EMS providers. If response times are being studied, then perhaps the study subjects are individual calls, or the individual patients. The research question and hypothesis will help to define who or what to study, but more refined inclusion and exclusion criteria will be required for each of these examples.

One final thing to consider in identifying the study population is the ethical implications of those decisions. Research ethics and the process of ethical review are covered in great detail in Chapter 9, but the researcher must consider some of those issues at this point. What are the ethical implications of including or excluding children? What are the ethical considerations of obtaining "informed consent" from patients in severe distress? Will students feel compelled to participate in a study because they think refusing to participate will affect their grade? Is it appropriate to manipulate EMS system characteristics when individual patients will not have the opportunity to consent to or reject those manipulations? These are not insurmountable issues, but they must be considered during the process of identifying the study population.

IDENTIFYING THE SETTING FOR THE STUDY

In addition to identifying the study population, the researcher must clearly define the setting in which the study will be conducted. This is important because many factors about the setting could affect the results. In the end, the study is really a test of the hypothesis within a specific setting. A multistate study of cold-water drowning, for example, will likely have different results if the study is conducted in Minnesota, the Dakotas, and Montana than if it is conducted in Virginia, the Carolinas, and Tennessee.

Just as with identifying the study population, the researcher tries to choose the setting that will best support testing of the study hypothesis. Each factor about the setting, and that factor's potential influence on the study, must be considered. With the exception of tightly controlled laboratory research, it is nearly impossible to obtain a perfect setting. In fact, given the inconsistencies among communities, EMS systems, hospitals, and populations, there really isn't a perfect setting for any EMS research project. The researcher is trying to find the best possible setting for conducting a specific study testing one particular hypothesis.

For most EMS studies, the setting will simply be the EMS system or the community in which it is located. Since this is the environment to which the researcher has access, it by default becomes the setting for the study. Even when a study is conducted within one EMS system or one community, there may be factors about the setting that must be prospectively decided. In a study about IV success rates, the researcher may want to limit the setting to the emergency response agency and not include the inter-facility transport service. In a study about a teaching methodology, the researcher may want to limit the setting to the full-time day paramedic classes and exclude the part-time night classes. In a study about the impact of fire department first responders, the researcher may want to exclude those places that already have medical personnel on site, such as nursing homes, doctor's offices, and some industrial plants.

Whether the study occurs in one specific setting or several different locations, the researcher must define the specific characteristics of the setting. These attributes will have to be reported along with the results so that others can decide how well the setting for the study relates to the EMS environment in general, and to their specific EMS system. What is the size of the city or cities where the study is being conducted? Is this a rural study, an urban study, or both? Is the community primarily an affluent one, or is it impoverished? How does the EMS system operate? Is it a full-time paid system? Does it incorporate a tiered response? How many responses does it have each year? These are just a few examples of the seemingly nitpicky details that the researcher must be able to identify. All of these things might affect the implementation and results of a study.

DECIDING WHAT DATA TO COLLECT

Deciding what data to collect will be as simple or as complex as the study question itself. Complicated hypotheses require a larger number of data points, while simple, specific hypotheses require fewer data points. For example, the hypothesis, "A patient's hemodynamic status predicts outcome," would require collection of data reflecting several variables. Hemodynamic status could be represented by level of consciousness, respiratory rate, heart rate, blood pressure, or dozens of other assessment findings. Outcome could mean a change in vital signs, an improvement in level of consciousness, discharge from the emergency department or admission to the hospital, survival, or neurologic function. Clearly, a great number of data would have to be collected to test this broad, poorly defined hypothesis. The more specific hypothesis, "Patients with heart rates of less than 50 are more likely to die than those with heart rates greater than 50," would require only two primary data points: heart rate and whether the patient died.

There are three types of variables that the investigator must consider. *Independent variables* are those things that the researcher wants to study—the study factors. *Dependent variables* are the things the researcher thinks might change or vary as a result of the independent variables. *Confounding variables* are things that the investigator is not really interested in, but that might somehow affect the study.

Independent variables are sometimes called *predictor variables*. They are usually identified, at least to some extent, by the hypothesis. In the examples above, hemodynamic parameters and heart rate would be independent variables. In experimental studies, the independent variable is the thing the researcher manipulates—the intervention. In a clinical study, whether a patient received the study drug or a placebo is an independent variable. In an educational study, whether a student was taught in a classroom or via distance learning might be an independent variable. In a systems study, whether a dispatch center has enhanced 911 capability or a noncomputerized facility using seven-digit phone numbers could be an independent variable.

Dependent variables are also called *outcome variables*. Like the independent variables, the dependent variables should be identified by the hypothesis. For example, the hypothesis for a clinical study of cardiac arrest patients should identify whether return of a pulse or survival to hospital discharge is the outcome of interest. In an educational study, test scores or student satisfaction might be outcome variables. In systems research, cost effectiveness or improved response times might be dependent variables.

Confounding variables are those things that might affect the study, but are not of particular interest to the investigator. One reason to conduct randomized trials is so that these confounding variables get evenly distributed, by chance alone, among all subjects. Unfortunately, sometimes the confounding variables, by chance alone, don't get evenly distributed. Consider a study comparing the effect of bystander CPR on survival from cardiac arrest in which the results show that more patients who received bystander CPR lived than those who did not. Now, consider what those results would mean if, just by chance, 18 percent of the patients in the bystander CPR group were in asystole, but 84 percent of the patients in the no-bystander CPR group were in asystole. Is the difference in survival really due to the bystander CPR? We already know that patients in asystole are less likely to be resuscitated than patients with a shockable rhythm. The patient's cardiac rhythm is a confounding variable.

Sometimes confounding variables can be eliminated during the process of defining the inclusion and exclusion criteria for patients, but that's not always possible. The patient's family history of heart disease might also be a confounding variable in a cardiac arrest study, but that information might not be immediately available at the time the patient is enrolled in the study. The researcher doesn't collect the confounding variables in order to study their influence or effect. They are collected so the researcher can identify potential differences among the study participants, and they are reported so the reader can consider how they impact the study's results.

Even when a study has a simple, specific hypothesis, the researcher is often faced with hundreds of potential independent, dependent, and confounding variables. For most researchers, the typical gut reaction is "more is better." The common notion is "If I have the data and don't use them, that's OK, but if I don't collect the data and then need them later, I'm in trouble." This isn't entirely illogical, but it can lead to great problems. An overabundance of data is as useless as no data—it muddies the waters. The process of determining which data points to collect is very similar to the process of refining the research question: Be as specific as possible. The independent and dependent variables should be those specified by the hypothesis, or those that are directly related to the hypothesis. Only those confounding variables that experience or previous studies suggest could impact the study should be collected. Otherwise, the researcher conducting a nationwide study of IV success rates might end up collecting the altitude at each study site "just in case it's a confounding variable." It's up to the investigator to draw the line somewhere, and in most cases less is more.

DECIDING HOW TO RECORD THE DATA

Once the researcher has identified the variables to be collected, the manner in which they'll be recorded must be determined. This is another instance in which the researcher must balance the concepts of "more is better" with "less is more." For example, if hypotension is one of the variables to be collected, should the researcher collect the actual blood pressure or simply record whether or not the patient was hypotensive? A space on a data collection form such as

Hypotension   Yes   No

in which the data collector circles the appropriate response, makes for easier data collection and data management, but it doesn't provide as much information as

Blood pressure   _____ / _____

The yes/no method also assumes that the people collecting the data and the study investigators all have the same definition for hypotension. To be certain, the researcher should probably specify a cutoff value for hypotension in the study protocol.

Another example would be a study in which the outcome variable is the presence or absence of shock. Does the investigator collect

Shock   Present   Absent

or

Blood pressure   _____ / _____
Pulse   _____
Diaphoresis   Yes   No
Altered mental status   Yes   No

and so on? These may seem like nitpicky issues, but each and every one of them will influence how the data are collected, how easy it is to collect data, the accuracy of the collected data, the way in which the data are analyzed, and the ability to control for confounding variables. There are no right or wrong approaches. It is up to the investigator to determine the method of data measurement that best suits the given study.

DEVELOPING THE EXPERIMENTAL PROTOCOL

It is only after the researcher has determined who the subjects will be, the setting in which they will be studied, the variables that will be collected, and how the variables will be measured that the actual experimental protocol can be designed. This is the step-by-step process for actually conducting the study. This is also the one place where more really is more. The protocol should be as detailed as possible to ensure that the study is implemented precisely as it was designed.

The researcher must first decide how subjects will be identified and enrolled in the study. Who the subjects are and where they will be studied has already been determined, but the process for enrolling them must be described. Will the paramedic at the scene determine whether or not a specific patient is enrolled? Or, will the paramedic make radio contact with a researcher or a base station physician to determine if the patient is eligible? Once the subject is identified, how will consent be obtained? If the research is conducted in a classroom, will students be able to withhold consent without standing out from the rest of the class? If a systems study involves chart reviews, and the researcher comes across one of his or her own charts, how will that situation be handled?

If the study involves the allocation or randomization of subjects to an intervention or control group, how will that be accomplished? Some common ways for allocating or randomizing patients include using an alternating-day approach, having the base station physician perform the allocation on a case-by-case basis, or stocking the ambulance with sealed envelopes that contain the randomization information. Whether one of these or some other method is used, the process must be clearly defined in advance.

Another important issue is whether the subjects will know which study group they are in. Will the paramedic, the instructor, or the system administrator know? Will the researcher know? While blinding everyone involved in the study makes for the purest science, it may not be practical—and in some cases it may be unethical. Who will and will not be blinded, how blinding will be maintained, and how the ethical concerns related to blinding will be addressed must all be described in the study protocol.

In an experimental study, the intervention must be strictly described. Exactly what will be done? How will it be done? A study evaluating the pain associated with starting an IV might want to go so far as to specify that the nondominant upper extremity will be used, or even to identify the specific brand and size of IV catheter. An educational study of a specific curriculum will have to define the curriculum in detail. (When reporting such a study, the curriculum does not necessarily need to be included in the report. It can be referenced or added as an appendix.) A system study might have to describe the 911 call-taking and dispatching procedure in great detail.

The protocol will also have to describe exactly how data will be collected and recorded. Much of this will have been decided during the process of determining which variables to collect and how they should be structured. Still, the protocol is the place for specifics. If the blood pressure needs to be recorded exactly 5 minutes after administration of a study drug, that should be spelled out in the protocol. The protocol may even need to specify that the blood pressure will be auscultated, not palpated. If data about student performance on a skills examination are being recorded, the method of observation and the criteria for each task must be specified. Can the student simply say "I would check the pulse," or must it actually be demonstrated? If a study requires the subjects themselves to record data, for example on a survey or on a pain scale, the protocol will have to describe precisely what instructions those subjects will receive.

The researcher should also try to anticipate problems in the data collection process and to plan for as many of those potential problems as possible. A study about immobilization published in *Prehospital Emergency Care* illustrated the difficulties of performing EMS research.[6] Originally, 48 people volunteered for the study, but only 39 completed the process. One person couldn't breathe while lying down; three volunteers were excluded because they "couldn't follow instructions"; four subjects "wanted to have their turn before others, and when they couldn't, withdrew their permission"; and data from one subject were lost when a machine ran out of recording paper. The data for approximately one-fifth of the subjects in the study were lost because of "problems."

The types of problems the researcher should anticipate depend on the study type and the study question. How will a survey study deal with subjects who cannot read? Will they be excluded from the study? Will someone read them the survey? Will they be asked to do the best they can? If a student drops out of a class in which a research project is being conducted, will all of the data collected on the student then be excluded? Will only the data collected so far be used, or will the investigator ask the student to complete the study even though he or she will not be completing the class? If the researcher is studying employee turnover rates in different systems, how will changes in management personnel or an unusual mass casualty incident affect those data, and how will those problems be addressed?

This is not to suggest that investigators should "what-if" about everything, but they should contemplate those problems that might reasonably be expected, and they should have a plan for responding to those issues. Again, there are no right or wrong answers in this process, but the researcher will have much greater success if these possibilities are addressed ahead of time.

TRADE-OFFS

The entire research process, and particularly the development of the methodology, is a series of trade-offs. Increasing the scientific nature of the study might make it more complicated; making the study easier to conduct might make the results less valid or less applicable to other settings. In some cases, a statistically significant outcome will be achievable, even though the results will not be clinically significant. Conversely, designing the study so that the results have clear clinical impact might affect the statistical significance. Conducting a large, multicenter trial that enrolls thousands of patients might produce a more sound conclusion, but it will also require more time, more energy, and more money. The researcher must decide— usually by looking back to the original question and hypothesis—what is necessary to make the study successful.

SUMMARY

It's not possible within this book, let alone this single chapter, to describe in detail every possible methodology for conducting every possible study. Each study is unique, and the methodology must be tailored to that study. It is up to the investigator to determine the most appropriate methodology for any given study. In developing the methodology, the researcher must consider several key components. Many of those components will be dictated, at least in part, by those steps in the research process that have already been completed. The overall research topic, the results of the literature search, the specific question and hypothesis, and the type of study to be conducted will all influence the study methodology.

In designing the methodology, the researcher must identify the study population, including inclusion and exclusion criteria. He or she must also identify the setting for the study and the specific characteristics of that setting, as well as decide what data to collect and how to record the data. The study protocol, detailing each step in the actual experiment, must be determined. It should include the process for allocating or randomizing subjects, the method of blinding (if any), and precise instructions on performing any research interventions. Finally, the researcher should anticipate problems in the study and try to develop strategies for addressing those problems when they occur.

In the end, the final methodology will be a compromise between rigid science and practicality, between comprehensiveness and available resources, and between clinically relevant and statistically significant endpoints. There is no perfect methodology.

A Typical Experience
Part 5: Developing the Methods

Mary and Tom had reserved the small meeting room at the main EMS station for the entire afternoon. Mary pushed one of the two tables in the room up against the wall and started setting up the coffee maker, while Tom stacked up all of the extra chairs, leaving just the four they'd need for the meeting. He put two on either side of the remaining table. They had copies of all of the articles Mary had found during the literature search, a copy of the EMS protocols, and a legal pad and pen for each person. Tom spread those out on the table.

"I guess we're ready, Mary. Tell me again why we're making such a big production out of this. And please tell me again why you invited Timmy."

"I just figured it was easier for us to all work on this together, instead of you and me doing it and then having Dr. Walsh tell us to change a bunch of stuff. I also figured Timmy would have something to say about this sooner or later, so we may as well get him in on it from the start. He's done these studies before, so I'm hoping he'll actually be helpful."

"Dreamer."

Mary sat down at the table and took one of the legal pads. She began writing:

Pt. Population
    Inclusion criteria
    Exclusion criteria
Setting
Experimental Protocol
    Identifying subjects
    Consent
    Randomization
    Interventions
Data Points/Data Forms
    Who collects
    How to collect
Analysis

"What am I missing, Tom?"

He read down the list. "I think that's it. I'm sure we'll think of more specific things as we go along, but that should get us moving in the right direction."

"Hey there," Dave Walsh said as he walked into the room. "I guess this is the right place, huh?"

"This is it." Mary walked over and shook his hand. Tom nodded a silent hello from across the room. "Timmy should be here any—"

"Speak of the devil!" Timmy exclaimed, standing in the doorway with his arms held out and his palms turned upward, as if to say "ta-da." "Hi, doc; Tom."

"Hi, Timmy. What do you guys want to drink?" Tom offered, walking toward the coffee maker.

Dave declined. "I'm good for now."

"I'll just have coffee. Black," Timmy said as he walked over to join Tom, who was pouring coffee into a "World's Best Paramedic" mug. Tom took a sip out of the cup and passed the pot to Timmy. "Here you go."

"So, what are we doing here?" Dave asked as they gathered around the table and pulled up their chairs.

Mary took the lead. "Well, we need to figure out a study design for this chest pain and aspirin study. I thought it would be best if we all worked on it together. We need you to make sure we don't do anything that's medically stupid, and we figured Timmy could help us out a lot since he's done these kinds of studies before." She kicked Tom's ankle under the table to make sure he stayed quiet. "I've kind of listed out the main points here," she said, pointing to the list on the legal pad. "I thought we could just work through each of these in order. I'm not sure we have to get every single detail down today, but I'd like to have a pretty clear idea of how we're going to pull this off."

Dave pulled the list over where he could see it. "OK. This looks reasonable. Let's start with the patients. Chest pain, right?"

"That's right," Tom said. "In our hypothesis we said, 'patients treated under the cardiac chest pain protocol.' We don't want to get the people with pulled muscles or blunt chest trauma."

"Why don't you just say, 'patients with cardiac chest pain'?" Timmy asked.

"We thought about that," Mary replied, "but we don't have any way to know whether someone's chest pain is *really* cardiac pain. It's the same reason we didn't say 'MI patients' specifically. There's no way to know that for sure in the field."

Timmy pursued the point. "Could you say '*suspected* cardiac chest pain'?"

Mary kicked Tom again just to be safe. "Sure, I guess, if you think that sounds better. I don't really care how we say it, as long as we get all of the patients who get treated under the cardiac chest pain protocol."

Dave decided to intervene. "I think Mary's right. How we word it isn't so important today, as long as we all agree on what we're doing. Let's not get too bogged down here. What's next?"

"Should we do the specific inclusion and exclusion criteria?" Mary asked.

"Yeah, we should probably work through at least some of that. Tom, Timmy, what do you guys have in mind?"

"Well," Timmy wrapped his arms across his chest and began to tip back in the chair, "clearly you have to exclude patients who are allergic to aspirin."

"Yep." Mary tore off a sheet from one of the pads and began to make a list.

"What about people who already take an aspirin every day?" Tom asked.

"Right now," Dave interjected, "isn't the protocol to go ahead and give them more aspirin anyway?"

"It doesn't really say one way or the other in the protocol," Tom explained. "I think that's what most people do, though. Otherwise they'd have to call in and get permission not to."

"Then let's keep them in the study." Dave offered. "I'd rather not have to rewrite the chest pain protocol just to get this research done."

"Should we have a specific age limit? Say, nobody under 35, or 30?" Tom was trying to be helpful.

"We normally don't treat younger people with the chest pain protocol, unless we really believe it's cardiac," Timmy replied.

"That's true," Tom admitted. "Well, are there other contraindications we should think about, other than aspirin allergy?"

"Now I think you're on the right track," Dave said encouragingly. "Think about stuff that would knock people out of the study even after they started the chest pain protocol, rather than thinking about what would keep them out of the chest pain protocol to start with. Allergies, known bleeding disorders . . ."

"Sometimes patients just refuse to take the aspirin," Tom added.

"And sometimes the paramedics just forget to give it!" Dave grabbed Tom's shoulder and shook it reassuringly. Tom smiled, but pulled away.

"Actually," Mary offered, "I'm not sure about patients refusing, but if we're going to do an 'intention to treat' analysis—or at least try to—I don't think the paramedic forgetting should be an exclusion."

"I guess that will depend on how we do the randomization," Dave agreed. "You're right, once they're randomized to get aspirin or not, whether they actually get it isn't really the issue. You're really studying whether including aspirin in the chest pain protocol makes a difference, not whether aspirin itself works."

"I'm not sure I understand that, doc." Timmy had tipped his chair forward onto all four legs and was leaning on the table. "We want to see the difference in patients who do and don't get aspirin. If the paramedic forgets, why wouldn't the patient go in the no-aspirin category?"

"It is kind of complicated, but it's a pretty basic research principle that you should analyze patients in the group they're randomized to, regardless of what actually happens." Dave took one of the legal pads and began to draw out a flowchart. "I can show you a small example of why."

"Well, I'll take your word for it." Timmy didn't like the idea of getting a lesson—any kind of lesson—from the medical director while his co-workers were looking on. "We don't have to spend time on that now."

Dave sensed Timmy's uneasiness. "To be honest, a lot of doctors have a hard time understanding 'intention to treat' analysis. It took me a long time to get it straight myself." He hoped that helped.

"Let's keep moving." Tom wanted to wrap this up before 4:00. He had a 4:30 tee time he hadn't told Mary about. "So the setting is easy. That's our EMS system. I know we'll have to describe it in detail at some point, but for now what else do we need to say?"

"We'll need to include our emergency department as part of the setting," Dave said. "The good news is that, since we're the official chest pain center, about 95 percent of all chest pain patients come to us. I guess I'm not sure if that's a setting issue or an exclusion criteria issue, but it would make it a lot easier to do this study if we only study patients who come to our facility."

"I'll call it setting," Mary decided. "It's the same issue as if someone is treated by an ambulance from a neighboring system during a mutual aid call. They're not part of the setting, either. I'll describe the setting as our system and Dave's ED. Patients transported by other EMS agencies or to other facilities are not in the setting, so they shouldn't be enrolled in the study."

"I'll bet you end up calling that an exclusion criterion." Timmy was over his uneasiness, at least enough to offer his opinion again.

Tom winced in anticipation of another kick from Mary. It didn't come, so he chimed in. "Maybe, Timmy, but we can deal with that when we have to write up the study. Right now it just matters that we're all agreeing that this is the way to do the study—whatever we call things."

"Alright." Dave didn't want the animosity between Timmy and Tom to escalate any more. "We've got a good handle on the population and setting, so let's dive into the study protocol."

It took almost a full two hours to work through the experimental protocol. To Mary's surprise, both Tom and Timmy were extremely helpful, and Dave pretty much just sat back and let them go. He did help them work through the consent process, reminding them that they could use the same approach that had been used for an albuterol study a few years ago.

They could read a standardized brief description of the study from a laminated pocket card and get verbal consent in the field. Then the formal written consent could be obtained at the emergency department. He did offer this caveat: "If this was a major intervention, the IRB might not let us do this. However, since we're really only talking about delaying an unproven intervention for 10 or 15 minutes, I don't think they'll have a problem with it."

The other place things got bogged down was with randomization. The group decided they had to figure out the randomization and interventions together. If they were going to compare aspirin to a placebo, they could randomize patients to get one or the other. If they were going to simply give aspirin in the field, or wait and give it in the ED, they could randomize the patients to either "now" or "later."

"I guess we should have thought about this when we decided on the type of study," Mary confessed.

"That's alright," Dave reassured her. "Thinking of this whole process as distinct sequential steps is a little artificial. Even if you had thought about this earlier, we'd still be trying to reconcile the interventions with the randomization scheme."

There were a lot of issues. If they did a placebo controlled trial, there would be the added expense of purchasing the placebo. It would be a better design because they could blind the patients and the paramedics to what they were getting or giving, but they'd probably have to break the blinding as soon as they got to the hospital so the ED staff would know whether or not the patient still needed aspirin. If they simply did "now" vs. "later," they wouldn't have the expense of the placebo, but there would be no way to do a blinded study.

Timmy offered an idea that seemed to make sense, enough so that Mary was actually glad she had included him in the meeting. "Why don't we package two doses together: one aspirin dose and one placebo dose. We can label them dose 1 and dose 2. Everyone gets dose 1 in the field, and everyone gets dose 2 in the ED. That way everyone gets both aspirin and placebo, and the only difference is whether they got aspirin early or aspirin later. The pharmacy can put codes on the packages to keep track of which ones have aspirin as dose 1 or dose 2, but they wouldn't need to break the code until the study was done and we started the analysis."

Tom was impressed. "Wow, Timmy, that's a great idea."

Working through the data collection process took just as long as figuring out the experimental protocol. Tom was irritated that he'd missed his tee time, but he was enjoying the process—although he would never admit that to Mary. He particularly enjoyed the discussions about what specific data points to collect, mostly because almost every time Timmy suggested something, Mary shot him down.

"We should collect the patients' rating of their chest pain, you know, on a scale of 1 to 10, and then repeat that at the emergency department to see if aspirin has any effect on their pain," was one of Timmy's suggestions.

"I understand your point, but we're really not studying whether aspirin affects chest pain. I don't want to get distracted by things that don't contribute to our specific interest." Mary was a woman with a mission now, and it was kind of fun to watch.

Timmy prefaced another suggestion with, "I don't mean this as a slam, Tom." Then he continued, "We really should track how many times the paramedic forgets to give aspirin and see if older paramedics are more likely to forget than younger ones."

"That's not our question either." Mary was focused. "You could easily do that as a QA study if you wanted to, but we're going to have enough trouble getting field paramedics to support this study without them thinking we're somehow examining them. I don't want to do anything that will make them suspicious of our motives."

They ended up with a relatively short list of data points. The field EMS people would have to record the date of the call; the patient's name, age, and sex; the duration of the pain; and the patient's home aspirin use, so they could compare the aspirin and placebo groups at baseline. They'd also have to record the code number from the medication package. The ED staff would have to complete the consent process and record whether the patient was admitted, discharged, or died; the name of the patient's primary care physician; and the patient's medical record number. It would be up to Mary and Tom, with a little help from Dave, to follow up and find out which patients got thrombolytics or went to the cath lab, and if any of the admitted or discharged patients eventually died. They decided to use 6 weeks as the cutoff point for follow-up.

Mary commented on that. "The ISIS-2 study used 5 weeks, and they only looked at vascular-related deaths. I'm not sure why they chose 5 weeks, but I don't think we're doing anything wrong by using 6. I guess someone might disagree with us looking at all deaths, regardless of cause, but I'm not sure how hard it will be for us to figure out the specific cause of death."

"I think 6 weeks and all-cause mortality are fine endpoints." Dave had been reasonably quiet for a long time, but he knew there were no right or wrong answers here and he didn't want the others to get bogged down in second-guessing themselves.

"At least the analysis will be pretty straightforward," Mary sighed, obviously growing tired. "I've talked to my neighbor some more, and she says simply using a two-by-two table to look at the proportion of patients who died in each group will be perfect. She said she could calculate a lot of statistical stuff; I didn't understand a bit of what she was saying. She is worried about how many patients we'll need for the study—I did get that much from her. We're supposed to meet next Tuesday to go over that."

"Is there anything else we need to do here today?" Timmy asked, growing bored.

"Nah, I think we're done." Mary began to gather her things. "I really appreciate you all staying here so late. I know this was a pain, but I think it's going to pay off for the study."

Chapter 8

Consulting a Statistician and Performing a Power Calculation

The next step in designing a study is to determine how many subjects need to be enrolled. This sample size is determined by doing a power calculation. The power calculation tells the researcher how many subjects should be enrolled to ensure that the study results are valid, and not just a result of chance. This is the first step in the process where the help of an experienced statistician is required; most researchers do not do this work on their own. As discussed later in the chapter, involving a statistician with this part of the project is essential, but it can also be helpful in all of the other steps as well.

SIGNIFICANCE

The concept of significance is extremely important in research. Suppose, for example, that a researcher compared the effectiveness of drug A and drug B in treating a terminal disease. The researcher might find that 73 percent of the patients who received drug A survived, and 74 percent of the patients who received drug B survived. Certainly, 74 percent is more than 73 percent, but is drug B really better than drug A? Is the difference between 74 percent and 73 percent significant?

STATISTICAL SIGNIFICANCE

In research, there are two kinds of significance: statistical significance and clinical significance. Statistical significance is a measure of how often the difference between data sets would occur just by chance alone. What if the drug A–vs.–drug B study were repeated 100 times? What if 99 of those studies found the drug A and the drug B survival rates to be exactly the same, and only 1 study found the 73 percent–vs.–74 percent difference? That one-time difference was probably just a fluke: It could happen by chance alone. But, if 99 out of the 100 studies found the 73 percent–vs.–74 percent difference, then it would appear that drug B really is 1 percent better than drug A.

Determining statistical significance is one way to limit the effects of chance on a study's results. Statistical tests tell the researcher how likely it is that the results of a study occurred simply by chance. Typically, a cutoff point of 5 percent is used to determine statistical significance. If the results of a study could happen by chance alone 5 percent of the time or more, that difference is not considered statistically significant. It's a pretty high standard: If the results would occur simply by chance 6 percent of the time, that means chance *would not* affect the results 94 percent of the time. Still, since the difference would occur by chance alone in more than 5 out of every 100 studies, that difference is not considered statistically significant.

The 5 percent cutoff value is also known as alpha (α). The alpha value is usually expressed using a decimal. An alpha of 5 percent is reported as an alpha of 0.05. Sometimes statisticians use other alpha values. There may be times when a researcher wants to be so certain that the difference is real that a cutoff, or alpha, of 1 percent is used. An alpha of 0.01 means the difference is accepted as significant if it would occur by chance no more than 1 out of 100 times. Although it happens rarely, there are also times when less restrictive alpha values are used. An alpha of 0.1, for example, would mean the difference would be accepted as significant if it would occur by chance no more than 10 out of 100 times.

The alpha value is one measurement of how much error a researcher will accept in a study. It is a measurement of alpha (or type I) error. Type I error means an error where the study finds a difference even though no real difference exists. Most studies accept a 5 percent chance of a type I error. The researcher plans the study knowing that the results could be wrong—that they could occur just by chance. But the study is powered (meaning it enrolls enough subjects) to ensure that there's less than a 5 percent chance of such an error occurring.

When statistical tests determine how likely it is that the differences between sets of data occurred by chance alone, they do so by calculating a *P* value. Like the alpha value, the *P* value is reported as a decimal indicating the likelihood of finding the results by chance alone. A *P* value of 0.03 means the results would happen by chance alone 3 out of every 100 times. The *P* value, however, is different from the alpha value. The alpha value is the cutoff level that the researcher sets when designing the research project. The *P* value is calculated by statistical tests. If the calculated *P* value is less than the predetermined alpha value, then the difference between the groups is said to be statistically significant. If the *P* value calculated by the statistical test is greater than the predetermined alpha value, the results are not statistically significant.

CLINICAL SIGNIFICANCE

It is important to remember that statistical significance is a mathematical construct and has little to do with practical difference. The researcher must be able to relate statistical significance to clinical relevance. Even if the difference between drug A and drug B is found to be statistically significant, the researcher (and the research reader) must still decide whether that difference is clinically relevant. Is a 1 percent reduction in mortality clinically significant? Perhaps it is. But what if the difference between the two drugs is one-tenth of 1 percent, and those results are statistically significant, too? Is saving 1 patient out of 1000 clinically significant? What about saving 1 out of 10000 patients?

There are rarely absolute right and wrong answers about clinical significance, and sometimes the questions are reversed. What if the difference in mortality is 20 percent, but the statistical tests say that difference could happen by chance alone 7 out of 100 times ($P = 0.07$)? The difference is not statistically significant, but would anyone question the clinical significance of a 20 percent reduction in mortality?

The trick to reconciling statistical significance and clinical significance is in designing the study. The EMS researcher must design the study in such a way that statistical findings are clinically relevant and clinically relevant findings result in statistical significance.

POWER ANALYSIS AND SAMPLE SIZE

Conducting a power analysis and determining the appropriate sample size is essential in creating a study that will have sound clinical and statistical findings. Performing the power analysis and determining the sample size is also one of the most difficult tasks for researchers. In order to conduct the power analysis, the researcher must predict what the results will be. Of course, if one knew what the results would be, it wouldn't be necessary to do the study. How can the EMS researcher be expected to predict the results?

First, the researcher must conduct a thorough literature search and be absolutely familiar with all of the science that has already been completed in the area of interest. This will help in predicting what the results will be. Then the researcher has to decide how big a difference between groups would be significant—how big a difference would be clinically relevant. This is known as the *effect size*. Then the researcher must decide what the alpha value will be and how strong the study should be. All of these pieces are plugged into a mathematical formula, and those calculations determine how many people need to be enrolled in the study in order to fulfill those requirements. This is complicated. Using the drug A/drug B example, the process may go something like this:

Drug A has been used for treating a terminal disease for the last 7 years. A paramedic has read every single research article about drug A, and he knows that the average survival rate for people who use it is 73 percent.

Now the EMT hears about a new medication, drug B. It appears that drug B might be better than drug A, and he wants to design a study to test that. He decides that if drug B is just 3 percent better than drug A, that would be clinically significant. It would, after all, save 3 more out of every 100 patients. He begins to design a study, and chooses to use the typical alpha value of 0.05, accepting up to a 5 percent chance that any differences discovered during the study could be simply due to chance alone.

Now, the researcher must decide how strong the study should be—how much power it will have. Just as there is the possibility of finding a difference due to chance alone, there is also the possibility of failing to find a difference even when one exists. This is called beta (β), or type II error. How big the chance of a beta or type II error is depends entirely on how many patients are enrolled in a study. Most of the time, studies are designed to have a power of 80 percent to detect the difference that is believed to be clinically relevant. In other words, if 100 drug A–vs.–drug B studies were conducted exactly the same way, 20 of those studies could fail to find the 3 percent difference in mortality, even if it really existed. Eighty of the studies would find the difference.

A study that has a 20 percent chance of failing to find a difference, even though that difference really does exist, might seem like a weak study. In fact, a power of 80 percent, or 0.8, is commonly accepted in medical research. Although it is possible to increase the power (or strength) of a study, to do so means the number of patients required for the study will also increase. For example, to have an 80 percent power of finding a 3 percent difference between drug A and drug B, 913 patients might be required in each group, for a total of 1826 patients. To increase the study power to 90 percent, as many as 1265 patients could be needed in each group, for 2530 total patients. To have a power of 99 percent—a nearly perfect study—might require 2329 patients in each group. Although a strong study is always desirable, it may be simply impossible to get such a large number of patients. As always, the researcher must balance the desire for a rigorous, strong study with the realities of resource and time constraints.

THE STATISTICIAN

By this point in the chapter, the EMS researcher should be convinced that the help of a statistician or epidemiologist will almost always be necessary for these calculations. This is a good thing! There is no shame in needing this help. In fact, most researchers should be ashamed of not seeking professional statistical help more often. A barber shouldn't be asked for legal advice, a mother shouldn't be asked for medical advice, and a paramedic, nurse or doctor shouldn't be asked for statistical advice. Ask a statistician.

THE STATISTICIAN'S ROLE

The role the statistician plays in a study will depend a lot on the researcher, the study, and the statistician. As the researcher gains experience, there may be certain parts of the research process that he or she feels comfortable tackling. However, there are statistical issues in each and every step, and the researcher should not hesitate to seek the advice of an expert.

Although the power calculation may be the first step in the research process in which the help of a statistician is required, the truth is that the help of a competent statistician can be invaluable in each and every step of the research process.

Identifying the Topic

Usually, the topics of EMS research projects relate to some clinical, educational, organizational, or systems issue. Most EMS research is problem-driven; it is undertaken in an effort to resolve a problem or answer a question. What could a statistician possibly know about EMS issues? Probably nothing. However, the statistician will know about problem solving in general. The statistician will know what is measurable and what is controllable. The statistician will bring an objective view to the process of identifying a topic.

An easy example of this process would be an attempt to answer the ultimate question: Does EMS make a difference? This is a great question. It is important. Everyone wants to know the answer. Unfortunately, it can't be answered in one study. The statistician can help to narrow the focus, and to pick a topic that is doable.

Reviewing the Literature

For the most part, the researcher may be on his or her own when it comes to reviewing the literature. The statistician can be helpful, though, in making sure the literature is understood. When papers are found that use statistical tests that the researcher doesn't understand, or when papers have results that seem to contradict the data, these should be reviewed with the statistician. There may be a perfectly good explanation for these inconsistencies, or there may be flaws in the paper. An expert's help will always be useful in sorting those things out.

Defining a Question and Formulating a Hypothesis

The statistician can also help in developing the question, formulating the hypothesis, and formulating the null hypothesis. It is important that the hypothesis really be about what the study intends to measure, and that the study measure what the hypothesis addresses. It would be inappropriate to hypothesize that a drug affects mortality and then measure respiratory rates. The statistician can bring an objective perspective to this process.

Determining the Type of Study and Developing the Methods

Perhaps the most frustrating thing for any statistician is when a researcher shows up with a bunch of data that have already been collected and says, "I need help analyzing this." The analysis of the data needs to be planned very early in the study. The analytical methods must be considered when determining the type of study to be conducted and when developing the study methodology. The person who is going to be responsible for analyzing the data should always be involved in the process of designing the study methodology.

The statistician can help in determining what kind of study to conduct, what data to collect, and how to collect the data in order to be able to answer the question.

If a statistician is not involved in this planning process, the researcher might end up with reams of data that are effectively useless.

Performing the Power Analysis

One of the key steps in designing the study is determining the number of patients, subjects, or observations needed. Although the researcher will have to make some educated guesses about what he or she expects to find, an educated guess is never a good way to decide on the sample size. Using a statistician will help to ensure that the study will have adequate power to differentiate between real findings and those that would occur by chance alone.

Obtaining IRB Approval

When a proposal is submitted to an ethics committee for approval, the committee will want to be sure that the study design is sound and that the research efforts will be successful. Having a statistician involved in each step of the research process will help to assure the ethics committee that the study is being designed appropriately. In fact, statisticians serve on many ethics committees. If a statistician has not been involved in the study design, and the study methodology has flaws, ethics committees are likely to withhold approval until those shortcomings are addressed.

Interacting with Providers

A statistician might be exactly the wrong person to try to convince EMS providers of the importance of a study. The statistician can help the researcher accomplish that, however. EMS providers will have concerns about the validity of the study, such as, "statistics can be used to prove anything," and unrealistic expectations about what is and what is not a significant finding. Although the EMS researcher will be the person who has to answer those questions, the statistician can help in preparing for the questions.

The Pilot Study

The pilot study provides a test run before investing the time and money necessary to complete a full-fledged research project. The pilot study should identify problems with the study methodology, the data collection tool, and the planned analysis. The statistician should review the results of the pilot study to be certain that the data that are generated can be analyzed in the way planned.

Collecting Data

The statistician will want to help design the data collection form. The process of transferring data from paper into statistical analysis software can be cumbersome. It can be made easier if the data form is set up in a way that facilitates keypunching of the data. There are several different ways of making the form user-friendly, and the method chosen for any individual study will depend on the type of data and the planned statistical tests.

Analyzing the Data

Here's where the statistician is most useful. Although the researcher may have a basic understanding of some of the tests available to analyze data, the statistician will know everything about those tests, and many other tests too. There may be reasons why the data, even though they involve mean blood pressures, cannot be analyzed using the t-test. There may be reasons why the chi-square (χ^2) test is not the best test for comparing the frequencies found in the data. It is the statistician's job to know the limitations of these tests, and to use appropriate alternative tests when they are indicated.

In the end, the statistician should be able to provide both descriptive statistics describing the data and analytical statistics evaluating the significance of the findings. The statistician should also be able to help the researcher understand the findings.

Reporting the Findings

When the study is finally complete and the researcher is preparing a paper for publication, he or she will want to have the statistician review the manuscript. The purpose of the paper is to describe to others exactly what was done and what was found. Remember that the job of statistics is to convey the data in standardized universal terms. The statistician will make sure that the statistical methods and results of the study are reported accurately and precisely. The statistician can also make sure that the results are presented in a way that is meaningful to the typical research reader.

WHERE TO FIND A STATISTICIAN

There really isn't any common source for statisticians. For EMS researchers who work with or near a medical school, finding a statistician should be easy. The medical school may employ statisticians expressly for the purpose of assisting in research. More often, there will be scientists working at the medical school, including physicians and bench scientists, who have developed expertise in statistics through their own research efforts. Because academic institutions place considerable value on research efforts, these statisticians and scientists affiliated with a medical school are often very willing to assist other researchers. They may, however, want something in exchange. The EMS researcher may have to agree to include their name on the author list, or might have to agree to be a subject in some other project they are conducting. By being creative, a deal can most likely be struck.

If the EMS researcher doesn't work closely with a medical school, he or she may also check with any local university. Although the researchers there may not have specific expertise in medical research, the statistical principles are constant across all sciences. Like medical schools, most universities place great value on research. A statistician or even a social sciences researcher at the local university may be motivated to help.

If there is no university in the area, the researcher might check with the community college. Not all community colleges place the same premium on research that universities and medical schools do. Still, there may be someone on the faculty at the local college who has an interest in research. If nothing else, there may be a statistics instructor who can help.

If all of the academic organizations have been exhausted, and a statistician still cannot be located, check with the city or county government. Most people who have completed graduate work in any field, including public administration or management, have had some exposure to research and statistics. Public health departments employ epidemiologists who, while they may not know the intricacies of the EMS environment, do know about bio-statistics. Even if the people in the local government offices don't feel qualified to help, they may be able to provide a referral to someone they know.

SUMMARY

The formulas involved in conducting a power analysis and sample size calculations are complex and beyond the scope of this book. There are complete texts on the subject, and there are also computer programs and Web sites that can perform the calculations for the researcher. The important concept here is that the power of the study, the sample size, and the magnitude of the difference that must be detected are all interrelated. Any change in one affects the others. Finding a balance that allows the researcher to find meaningful differences while controlling for the effects of chance is the art of determining the sample size. Although there are computer resources that can help with the process, the issues associated with power analyses and sample size can be complex.

While this is the first area in which the help of a professional statistician or epidemiologist is essential, it isn't the only step in which that help will be useful. Successful researchers will involve a statistician in every step of the research process. Doing so will improve the quality of any investigative effort.

A Typical Experience
Part 6: Consulting a Statistician and Performing a Power Calculation

Mary and Tom had been over the study design a dozen times in the three days since they met with Dave and Timmy. They felt like they had a fairly good grasp on what they wanted to do and how they were going to get things done. One of the things they were still unsure about, though, was how long it was going to take to complete the study. Once they had an estimated sample size, they'd have a better idea about that.

"Hi, Katie, this is my partner, Tom," Mary said by way of introduction. "Tom, this is my neighbor, Katie."

Katie stuck out her hand. Tom nodded, "Hi, nice to meet you."

Mary continued, hoping to ease the awkwardness, "We really appreciate you taking the time to meet with us. I know you're busy."

"Not a problem." Katie pulled two aluminum and black plastic chairs in out of the hallway and closed the door to her office. As Tom and Mary sat down, she went back to her desk and sorted through the piles of papers for a notepad. "Now, tell me again what it is you're trying to do."

"When we take care of people having chest pain," Mary said, "we always give them aspirin because it's supposed to reduce blood clotting. Clots in the arteries of the heart are the cause of a lot of heart attacks. The thing is, nobody knows whether giving aspirin in the ambulance is better than waiting until you get to the hospital."

"Is there any reason to think it would be worse to give aspirin in the ambulance?" Katie asked.

"Not really, but it just adds to things we have to get done in a short period of time. We already have to give oxygen, start an IV, monitor the heart, and give nitroglycerin. Plus the ambulance company has the added expense of supplying the aspirin. None of those are major things, but we just have this history in EMS of doing stuff without knowing if it makes any difference. We'd kind of like to change that."

"I guess that's not unreasonable." Katie reached over to her mouse and launched one of the applications on her computer. "So how do you think you'll measure whether aspirin makes the patient better?"

"We've looked at a bunch of literature on this. The thing that most of them measure is mortality. The evidence is pretty good supporting the role of aspirin. There's this one," Mary said, passing a copy of the ISIS-2 study to Katie, "that shows a reduction in mortality at 5 weeks. But it only looks at aspirin or no aspirin, not how soon the aspirin is given."

"What did they find?"

"Well, it's a little screwy, because they also had people getting clot-busting drugs. When they looked only at the effect of aspirin, they found 9 percent of patients who got aspirin died, compared to 12 percent of patients who didn't."

"Wow," Katie was surprised. "Around 10 percent of your chest pain patients actually die? That seems like a lot."

Tom spoke up, "That's a little misleading. Those were all patients having an MI—uh, a heart attack. Not all of our chest pain patients are actually having heart attacks, so our percentages should be lower."

"But," Mary added, "we don't have any way to know who's having a heart attack and who's not, so we have to treat them all the same."

"Well, let's work through this," Katie said. She picked up a pencil and flipped to a clean page on the notepad. "How many chest pain patients do you have in a year?"

"We have about 43,000 calls a year, and somewhere around 8 percent of them are for chest pain. At least that's what our annual report from last year says." Mary went on, "I'd guess that only about 1 in 5 is actually having an MI."

"OK," Katie was doing some quick calculations in her head. "Eight percent of 43,000 is about 3000 . . . no, 3500. Twenty percent of that would be 700. So you think you get about 700 true heart attacks a year?"

"It seems like a lot when you say it that way." Mary did her own calculations. "That's like 60 a month, or 15 a week. Do you think we really have that many, Tom?"

"I don't know. That's two, maybe three a day. That's probably a little high."

"Let's work through it this way." Katie pointed to Mary. "How many chest pain calls do you have on an average shift?"

"I don't know, I'd say usually at least one. Sometimes three, sometimes none."

"That's OK." Katie continued, "Now, how many other ambulances are staffed on any given shift?"

"It varies by time of day," Tom answered, "but I'd guess we usually have six or eight rigs on the streets."

"OK, so that would be—on average—seven chest pains per shift. Do you work 8- or 12-hour shifts?"

Mary and Tom answered in unison, "Twelves."

"So that's 14 chest pains a day, or about 100 a week. You said 1 in 5, or 20 percent, would be heart attacks, so that's 20 a week. So, if your estimates are right, even if only 15 percent are actually heart attacks, that would still give you close to 700 a year."

"We're killing more people than I thought we were," Tom said, feigning remorse.

"Now," Katie was still ciphering on her pad. "According to the paper you showed me, if they don't get aspirin, about 12 percent of those 700 people will die, or 84 a year. When you look at all of your chest pain patients, that means 84 out of the 3500 die each year. That's a pretty small percentage." She scribbled some more on the pad. "Let's see, that would be two . . . two and . . . well, about two-and-a-half percent. Since we're just using round numbers here, let's say 3 percent. If only 3 percent of your chest pain patients die without aspirin, it's going to be pretty hard to show a big improvement with giving it. You're going to need a lot of patients."

"How many is a lot?" Mary asked, unsure whether she really wanted to know.

"That depends. How big a difference do you think would be meaningful? Let's say you reduced the death rate from 3 percent to 2 percent. That would mean you'd have to treat 100 patients with aspirin to save 1 life; only 2 out of every 100 people would die instead of 3. If aspirin reduces the death rate from 3 percent to 1 percent, then you'd only have to treat 50 patients to save 1 life."

"I don't know," Mary said. "I think making 1 out of 100 patients better would be pretty good, but 1 out of 50 would be more impressive to the docs and other paramedics."

"It would be easier to find, too," Katie offered encouragingly.

"Alright, so if we go with 1 in 50, how bad is that?" Mary asked.

Katie clicked her mouse, and then punched some numbers into her computer. "Assuming you want a power of 0.8, and will use an alpha value of 0.05, then you'd need . . . let's see . . . 769 patients in each group."

"Just to make sure I have this straight," Mary asked, "that means if there really is a 2 percent difference in mortality, we'd find it 80 percent of the time? And we have a 5 percent chance of finding that difference just by dumb luck, even though it might not be a true difference?"

"That's right."

"Are we talking about chest pain patients or MI patients?" Tom asked.

"I did all this based on the chest pain numbers. Since you have no way of knowing if a patient is really having a heart attack, it doesn't make much sense to base the calculations on that."

"So we have to transport 1400 chest pain patients?" Tom asked, discouraged.

"Actually," Katie corrected his math, "a little more than 1500. I'd suggest you shoot for at least 800 per group—1600 patients—just to be safe. Invariably you'll lose some of them. The good news is, you've already told me you transport about 3500 chest pain patients a year, so you might be able to get this done in 6 months if you really work at it."

"Timmy's going to love this," Tom complained.

"He'll just have to get over it," Mary said matter-of-factly. "Katie, is it realistic to try to do this in 6 months?"

"Probably not. You'll be amazed by the number of patients that you'll miss. Remember, some of them will have exclusion criteria, there'll be some of your colleagues who'll just refuse to enroll patients, and even some of those patients who do get enrolled will have incomplete data. I'd suggest you try one of two approaches. Either decide you're going to collect data for a set period of time—I'd suggest at least 8 months, if not a year—or decide to just collect data until you get 1600 patients—whenever that is."

"Mary," Tom warned, "I told you, I'm retiring in 8 years."

"You *might* be done by then." Katie laughed.

"Well, at least we know what we're up against." Mary stood up. "Katie, thanks a lot. We'll be sure to get back with you about our data forms and stuff before we start the study. I know you want to review all that to be sure we've got everything right."

"Glad to do it." Katie stood up and shook Mary's hand.

Tom nodded, "Appreciate the help."

SECTION 4

INTERACTIONS WITH OTHERS

Chapter 9

Ethical Considerations and IRB Approval

Each research project raises a set of distinct ethical uncertainties. It is the responsibility of the researcher to acknowledge these ethical questions and to address them within the context of the regulations that guide the research process.[7-10]

Participation in any research project involves some measure of risk. The risk is relative to the invasiveness of the research protocol. The risk can be in the form of such things as physical harm from procedures, side effects of medications, or perhaps failure of an experimental treatment. Risks are not limited to studies of clinical interventions, however. Even a chart review places a subject at some measure of risk. The risk associated with a chart review can be in the form of psychological or social harm from a loss of privacy. All research—clinical, educational, or systems—involves some element of risk.

THE HISTORICAL BACKGROUND TO ETHICAL ISSUES

The need to protect human subjects from research risks has been repeatedly demonstrated throughout history. The Nuremberg tribunals following World War II exposed the heinous experimentation done by German physicians on prisoners in concentration camps. While these experiments may have provided some valuable information about the human body, they were done at a tremendous cost both to the individuals involved and to society. As a result of the Nuremburg investigations, it became evident that researchers must be guided by a formal code of ethics as it relates to human experimentation. The Nuremberg Code of 1947 became the first code for ethical conduct in the use of humans in experiments.

Yet, examples of unethical research practices are not limited to Nazi Germany, and such practices have persisted despite the Nuremberg Code and subsequent guidelines. Between 1928 and 1972, during experiments conducted by the U.S. Public Health Service and investigators at Tuskegee University, African American men who were infected with syphilis were studied in an attempt to explore the natural progression of the disease. The researchers never told these men that they were infected, and treatment was either withheld or minimized to ensure that the disease did indeed progress. When men in the study died, the researchers offered to pay for their burial in exchange for permission from survivors to perform autopsies. These studies did not stop until 1972, and were only stopped then because of the public outcry that occurred after the experiments were exposed in newspaper articles. Further, the Tuskegee experiments are not the sole blemish on the U.S. research record. The military's study of personnel exposed to radiation during nuclear bomb testing in Nevada and New Mexico and the testing of vaccines on mentally impaired children are just two of the many other examples of studies that have failed to comply with ethical standards.

Today's ethical guidelines include the Nuremberg Code, the Helsinki Declaration of 1964 (including amendments from 1975, 1983, and 1989), the Belmont Report, and guidelines from the World Health Organization.[7,11]

In understanding the importance of ethical constraints on research, it is imperative to realize that researchers do not set out to conduct unethical studies. The physicians in Nazi Germany, the investigators at Tuskegee, and the military researchers mentioned earlier all believed they were conducting meaningful, well-intentioned, worthwhile research. Most researchers undertake their projects with the true belief that their work is important. The difficulty is that most researchers—like all people—find it difficult to objectively evaluate their own efforts.

ETHICAL PRINCIPLES

It is not the intent of the ethical codes to preclude the conducting of research, but merely to require that the researcher reduce the risks of research as much as possible and protect the most powerless in society. There are three basic ethical principles that should guide the development of any research project: (1) respect for persons, (2) beneficence, and (3) justice. Adhering to these three principles will help to ensure that a study is ethical.

First and foremost is the principle of respect for persons. This requires that the researcher treat subjects as self-sufficient, self-directed individuals who should be actively included in determining their involvement in the research process. This goes beyond simply consenting to medical care. By its nature, research is outside of what most people would consider standard or routine care. Patients must have the opportunity to decline participation in research without fearing they are jeopardizing their access to care. Also, before agreeing to participate in research, subjects must understand the potential risks and benefits associated with the study. This is accomplished through the process of obtaining informed consent, in which patients, or research subjects of any kind, are informed of the study and agree to their participation in the project. Care must be taken not to treat subjects as merely sources of data, but as unique individuals without whom there would be no research.

The principle of beneficence states that research projects should be developed to provide valid, useful, and generalizable information. Studies that pose any risk to the subjects must do more than provide information that may be of theoretical value. Theoretical knowledge is built through nonhuman or nonexperimental research, including surveys, retrospective analyses, and laboratory experiments. Clinical trials are intended to evaluate interventions only after a thorough understanding of the topic has been achieved through earlier nonhuman, nonexperimental work. Beneficence also requires that the benefits of the research outweigh the risks assumed by the subjects. Subjects who volunteer must be protected by minimizing risks within the study. A study of an intervention that is expected to result in a 10 percent decrease in postoperative scarring but is also predicted to have a 3 percent increase in mortality would not meet this standard: The benefits do not outweigh the risks.

The third principle, justice, requires that all potential participants bear the risks and benefits of the project equally. All research subjects accept some risk for participation; however, no single group of individuals should share an undue amount of the risk. One specific aim of this principle is protecting vulnerable populations who may not realize they have the right to refuse participation or who might fear some sort of reprisal should they do so.

Justice also requires that no single group be excluded from a study. Studies that do not include all potential subjects, including women, children, and minority populations, must be able to justify the exclusion. Indeed, federal funding guidelines now require the inclusion of such people in government-funded research, unless there is a clear and compelling reason not to include them.

To some extent, the requirement to spread the risk over all populations can be met through a solid randomization scheme. For example, a study that includes women but allows treatment assignments to be determined by the attending physician carries the risk that physicians will preferentially assign more men to a given treatment group than women. This is not to suggest that physician scientists are intentionally unethical. Instead, the bias is likely to be a product of some underlying, unknown influence from their training or experience, and they are most likely not even aware of it. True randomization of treatment assignments would avoid the influence of such bias.

FEDERAL GUIDELINES

The Department of Health and Human Services (DHHS) has developed a set of regulations that ensure that clinical research is conducted in an ethical and safe manner.[8] These are federal guidelines that are subject to local interpretation and implementation; however, the institutions that conduct or support research activities require that all research adhere to these standards. These federal guidelines serve as the basis for the policies and procedures of the internal review boards for all major universities in the U.S. The DHHS research guidelines state that the risk posed to the individual subject should be minimized. Table 9.1 summarizes the seven major guidelines developed by the DHHS.

The DHHS guidelines also require that projects involving clinical interventions routinely evaluate collected data to protect current and future subjects from harm. This means that at preestablished times during the data collection phase someone

Table 9.1   Summary of U.S. Department of Health and Human Services Guidelines for IRB Approval of Human Research (from 45CFR46.111)

1: Risks to subjects are minimized.
2: The risks are proportional to the potential benefits.
3: Subject selection is unbiased and equitable.
4: Informed consent is sought from each subject.
5: Informed consent is documented.
6: Data are routinely monitored to ensure safety.
7: Confidentiality is adequately protected, and additional safeguards are included for vulnerable populations.

must review the data to identify any untoward results—for example, unexpected deaths, high rates of disability, significant complications, or other problems that could be a result of the project.

The data monitoring can be conducted by someone involved with the project, by someone from the funding agency, or by an independent data monitoring board. An independent monitoring board is necessary when it is important that the investigators and/or funding agency remain blinded to the study intervention and effects. The board can be established as a part of the study protocol, with a predetermined schedule for meeting and analysis of the data. If at any point the analysis reveals any serious negative effects of the project, the study must be stopped and the problems must be reported to the sponsoring agency.

THE INTERNAL REVIEW BOARD

An internal review board (IRB) is a group of experts from the fields of theology, sociology, psychology, medicine, and members of the general public that is tasked with protecting research subjects. IRB is a generic term; there are many different names for these review panels. The role of the IRB, however, is consistent. These individuals review all aspects of a proposed research project, including the methodology and the potential benefits to society if the project is conducted. They evaluate the risks to the subjects, the benefits to the subjects, and the safety measures in place to protect the subjects from harm. Their job is to ensure that all human research adheres to the principles of respect, beneficence, and justice.

No two IRBs are the same. They share a common set of policies and procedures as outlined by the DHHS, but how they interpret and implement those guidelines is entirely up to the institution. This can be frustrating to the researcher, especially when a project requires approval from more than one IRB, but this variability is actually critical to the function of the IRB. What is acceptable and/or reasonable is, in large part, a community standard, and communities differ from each other. What is reasonable in New York City is likely to be different from what is reasonable in a small, one-stoplight community. Indeed, what is reasonable in New York City may be different from what is reasonable even in Chicago.

Many researchers begrudge the IRB as an impediment to research. But, as discussed earlier, the IRB process is required to ensure that all human subject research is ethical. Despite the best of intentions, it is impossible for any researcher to objectively and completely evaluate the potential risks and benefits of his or her own research project. In truth, the IRB process often contributes significantly to a proposed project. The questions and suggestions raised by members of the IRB can be extremely helpful in improving the study question, hypothesis, design, or intended analysis.

THE IRB PROCESS

The typical IRB process involves submitting an application package to the IRB office. Each institution will have its own application requirements. An administrator will review this application to ensure that all of the information is provided, and to identify any obvious problems. The administrator will then forward the application to the IRB chair, and the proposal will also be sent to two or three peer reviewers. Then the entire IRB panel will review the IRB proposal along with the comments from the reviewers. If changes or revisions are necessary, the investigator will be notified and given the opportunity to address those issues. It is rare for an IRB to summarily reject a proposed project.

Not all proposals require full IRB approval. Studies can be exempt from IRB approval, or they can undergo expedited review. The types of research that qualify for exempt or expedited review are established by the DHHS guidelines, but, as with all IRB issues, these are subject to local interpretation.

The types of studies that may be exempt from IRB approval are listed in Table 9.2. However, investigators should always check the requirements of the local IRB, as these may be more stringent. Remember, an IRB must review every research proposal. Only the IRB can make a determination as to whether a project is in fact exempt. Usually the IRB chair or IRB administrator performs this review without full IRB review, but, like all things IRB, this varies from institution to institution.

Local IRBs can also establish which projects can undergo an expedited review. Expedited reviews usually involve the review by the administrator and/or IRB chair, along with peer review. The investigator makes whatever revisions the reviewers suggest, and the process is completed without review by the entire IRB panel. DHHS guidelines allow expedited review only in those studies that pose a "minimal risk" to subjects. The guidelines define minimal risk as that which could be encountered during daily life or the performance of routine medical or psychological testing.[8]

SUBJECT SELECTION

One specific question asked on most internal review board applications is about subject selection. If a specific subset of the population (such as children or the elderly) is necessary for the project, a detailed explanation is expected. When a research proj-

Table 9.2   U.S. Department of Health and Human Services List of Research Exempt from IRB Review (from 45CFR46.101)

(1) Research conducted in established or commonly accepted educational settings, involving normal educational practices, such as (i) research on regular and special education instructional strategies, or (ii) research on the effectiveness of or the comparison among instructional techniques, curricula, or classroom management methods.

(2) Research involving the use of educational tests (cognitive, diagnostic, aptitude, achievement), survey procedures, interview procedures or observation of public behavior, unless: (i) information obtained is recorded in such a manner that human subjects can be identified, directly or through identifiers linked to the subjects; and (ii) any disclosure of the human subjects' responses outside the research could reasonably place the subjects at risk of criminal or civil liability or be damaging to the subjects' financial standing, employability, or reputation.

(3) Research involving the use of educational tests (cognitive, diagnostic, aptitude, achievement), survey procedures, interview procedures, or observation of public behavior that is not exempt under paragraph (2) of this section, if: (i) the human subjects are elected or appointed public officials or candidates for public office; or (ii) Federal statute(s) require(s) without exception that the confidentiality of the personally identifiable information will be maintained throughout the research and thereafter.

(4) Research involving the collection or study of existing data, documents, records, pathological specimens, or diagnostic specimens, if these sources are publicly available or if the information is recorded by the investigator in such a manner that subjects cannot be identified, directly or through identifiers linked to the subjects.

(5) Research and demonstration projects which are conducted by or subject to the approval of Department or Agency heads, and which are designed to study, evaluate, or otherwise examine: (i) Public benefit or service programs; (ii) procedures for obtaining benefits or services under those programs; (iii) possible changes in or alternatives to those programs or procedures; or (iv) possible changes in methods or levels of payment for benefits or services under those programs.

(6) Taste and food quality evaluation and consumer acceptance studies, (i) if wholesome foods without additives are consumed or (ii) if a food is consumed that contains a food ingredient at or below the level and for a use found to be safe, or agricultural chemical or environmental contaminant at or below the level found to be safe, by the Food and Drug Administration or approved by the Environmental Protection Agency or the Food Safety and Inspection Service of the U.S. Department of Agriculture.

ect proposes to include vulnerable populations, such as prisoners, children, or fetuses, the protocol is given a more intensive review. The principle of justice, as defined earlier, clearly states that no one single group should shoulder the greatest amount of risk, unless this is the target audience for the study results. That's not to say that it is never appropriate to target specific populations, only to say that doing so must be justified. For example, a study of triage to a pediatric specialty center would not be expected to enroll adult patients, and a study of testicular cancer would not be expected to enroll women.

Subjects who are going to be enrolled in a research project should consent to that participation. Informed consent is based on the principle of respect for persons. In the informed consent process, it is expected that the researcher will provide the potential subject with all relevant information so the individual can adequately understand and judge the risks and benefits of participating in the project. The consent document given to the subject must include an overview of the nature of the project and a description of the procedures involved in the research project, including both invasive and noninvasive procedures. The potential risks and benefits associated with participation must be detailed, as must the project timeline. The document must also include a description of the types of data that will be collected, and must describe how the data will be managed, who will have access to the data, and how confidentiality will be maintained. Most importantly, the document must assert that participation is completely voluntary, and that choosing to participate or not participate will not change the level of care to which the subject is entitled. While most discussions about consent in medical research presume the subject to be a patient, the rules are the same when the subjects are students, volunteers, members of a community, or any human beings.

In some populations, obtaining consent can be problematic. If the subject is incapacitated, underage, or incarcerated, the rules of informed consent are slightly altered.

For patients who are mentally incapacitated, it may be acceptable to obtain consent from a surrogate or proxy. That surrogate, however, must act in the best interest of the subject. Thus, a mentally incapacitated patient's physician, who is also a colleague of one of the investigators, would not be an appropriate surrogate. Mentally incapacitated patients may include the mentally ill, who typically have an appointed guardian, or those who are temporarily or newly incapacitated, such as people who have just suffered a stroke. For studies involving subjects who are acutely incapacitated, the next of kin may be able to act as a surrogate. Whatever the strategy for obtaining consent from a surrogate, it must be evaluated and approved by the IRB prior to study implementation. Such strategies can be expected to undergo close scrutiny.

In the case of prisoners, the individual may be able to consent, but the researcher must recognize the potential for undue influence over such people. Prisoners may perceive that their participation in the study might enhance their chances for early release or parole, or that it at least might improve the way prison officials treat them. Such perceptions, whether accurate or not, may amount to undue influence. Thus, an IRB may not allow the enrollment of prisoners and instead require that another comparable population be used in order to protect those who may feel pressured to participate. It is not appropriate for the custodians of prisoners—wardens, guards, etc.—to consent on the prisoners' behalf.

In the case of a minor, consent must be obtained from both a parent or legal guardian and the child. While children do not have the legal standing to provide consent on their own, they do—particularly as they get older—have the ability to understand issues relating to their care, and should have a voice in those decisions. The researcher should explain the study to both the parent and the child, and both should have the opportunity to agree to or decline participation. In cases where the child is too young to understand the issues, or is for some other reason not able to make a reasonable judgement about participation, the parent may provide consent for the child's participation without the child's consent. Technically, this is known as *parental assent*.

In emergency medicine and emergency medical services, medical care is sometimes provided under implied consent. That implied consent, however, does not generally extend to participation in research. The IRB can, however, approve a waiver of consent in such circumstances. Under a waiver of consent, patients are treated according to an established protocol that has been approved by the IRB. The requirements for waiver of consent are the subject of much discussion, and their interpretations will vary from community to community. The waiver of consent provision may be used when subjects are comatose or incapacitated and thus unable to provide informed consent, when a study does not alter the standard of care and the risk to the subjects is minimal, or when the study involves an exempted or expeditable protocol.

The consent process, much like the IRB process, is sometimes viewed as troublesome and obstructionist. Researchers typically believe they have the best interest of society at heart, and find it difficult to subject themselves to a process that suggests they might not be completely ethical. One way to come to terms with these beliefs is to look at the issue from the patient's perspective.

Consider, for example, a study of survival after defibrillation by laypeople using automatic defibrillators. The defibrillation has been done; the subject has survived and is now in the hospital. No further intervention is planned. Why should a researcher have to obtain consent to follow the patient's hospital course? Yet, if one imagines oneself as that patient, certainly one would want to know whether the physician overseeing one's care had an interest in—and possibly a bias about—whether or not one would survive to hospital discharge!

ANIMAL RESEARCH

The use of animals in medical research is a complex issue that is filled with emotion for advocates on both sides of the issue. Animal rights activists charge that the use of animals is cruel. Supporters of animal research point out the scientific advances that have come from such work. Whether one chooses to participate in animal research must, at this point, remain a personal decision.

The fact is that animals cannot provide informed consent. Thus researchers must provide adequate safeguards to ensure that animals used in research receive appropriate care, food, and shelter, and that they are not subjected to cruel or unusual pain or suffering. Institutions that participate in animal research utilize an ethics review process to ensure that all animal research is performed in as humane a process as possible.

Many of the questions that are asked of the researcher considering an animal study are similar to those asked of researchers conducting human studies, and the process for approval of animal research is very much the same as that for human experimentation. The board that reviews animal research will consist of many of the same individuals as that for human research, with the addition of a veterinarian. It is the job of the veterinarian to review the methodology to ensure that the animal receives appropriate anesthesia, pain relief, and care during the course of the experiment. The veterinarian, along with the rest of the committee, will also review the study to make sure that the animal being used is an appropriate model, and that there is not some other way to conduct the research without using animals. As with the human IRB, the role of the animal use committee is not to make research difficult or impossible, but to ensure that any animal research is ethical and humane.

GETTING ETHICS APPROVAL

The actual system for gaining review and approval by an ethics panel—whether for human or animal research, whether expedited or full review—will vary from institution to institution. Investigators must be completely familiar with the requirements of the institution in or with which they work. Most IRB and animal use committees have written guidelines and standardized submission forms that they will provide to researchers. Knowing the local requirements is essential in planning a successful research project.

The researcher's relationship with the ethics board should not be adversarial. Indeed, the IRB review process can be extremely helpful in ensuring that a study will be successful. Investigators should try to get to know the IRB chair and administrator. Meeting with them to discuss planned projects before actually submitting the application is always a good idea, and can help the researcher to anticipate problems and issues. Rather than viewing the ethics process as a hurdle that must be overcome, successful researchers learn to use the process to improve their studies.

The time it takes for ethics review will also vary by institution. In larger institutions the IRB or animal use committee will meet more frequently, and thus the process may be faster. The IRB guidelines usually describe the process and the time needed, and investigators should plan appropriately. It is not acceptable to start data collection while awaiting IRB approval. Completing the IRB process—even if it means simply going through the formality of having a project approved as exempt—is a prerequisite to study implementation.

The researcher should probably expect a request for revisions to the protocol. While revisions are not always required, the researcher must plan for them in the research timeline. If the project is approved without requiring revisions, the investigator has the opportunity to get ahead on the timeline. If, on the other hand, the researcher does not include time for protocol revision in the project timeline, he or she will almost certainly end up behind schedule. Again, don't view the request for revisions as an obstacle or a nuisance; think of it as part of the process of perfecting the study.

SUMMARY

Research involving human subjects must conform to a variety of federal guidelines designed to protect individuals and animals from undue harm. These guidelines include minimization of risk, equitable subject selection to protect the vulnerable, the assurance of confidentiality in the data collection and reporting process, and obtaining informed consent when feasible.

Nothing should be higher than the standards that researchers set for themselves. All research should be ethical and safe for potential participants. Establishing high personal standards is an excellent way to ensure ethical research projects. But all researchers must remain aware of the difficulty in assessing their own conduct, keeping in mind examples like the Nazi experimentation and the Tuskegee trials.

Because of the difficulty in objectively judging one's own actions, the institutional review board process must be an integral part of the development of a research project. The IRB provides safeguards to protect subjects from harm—whether physical, social, psychological, or other. The IRB is the research gatekeeper. No research on human subjects should be conducted without its approval.

A Typical Experience
Part 7: Ethical Considerations and IRB Approval

"This IRB stuff is getting complicated," Tom complained. "Why didn't you give me something easy to do?"

Mary had her trump card all ready. "Would you rather work on getting Timmy to help with the study?"

"You know, this IRB stuff isn't so complicated after all," Tom laughed. "All I have to do is get your friend Katie's college IRB to approve the study, Dave's hospital IRB to approve it, and apparently the EMS advisory council has to OK it too."

"Can you at least use the same format for all of them?" Mary asked.

"Nope. That would be too easy. The only good news is that both the community college and the advisory council have said that as long as the hospital IRB approves the project, they shouldn't have any problems with it."

"When do you expect to hear from the hospital?"

"Already have," Tom said. "Dave helped me with all the issues about respect for individuals, beneficence, and justice, so they were OK with that. They accepted the protocol. They just had some questions about the consent process, and they want us to do an interim analysis after the first 400 patients in each group. If there's a big difference at that point, they'll want us to stop the study."

Mary looked up. "What was wrong with the consent process?"

"Nothing major. They felt like the way we worded the stuff for the verbal consent would have pressured patients to agree to be in the study. We had put:

" '. . . if you agree to participate, you will receive one medication now and one when you arrive at the hospital. Neither you nor I will know which medication is real and which one is placebo. If you choose not to participate, you will receive only the standard care for your condition.'

"They felt like saying '*only* the standard care' makes it sound like that is less than what they'd get if they entered the study. They thought patients might agree to participate thinking that would give them a chance of getting more than the standard care. They just want us to take out the word *only*."

"That's not so bad." Mary was relieved. "I was afraid they were going to require us to do the entire written consent process in the ambulance."

"Apparently they talked about that. Dave was at the meeting, and he explained to them that if they did that we would be at the hospital before we could even get through the consent document. He told them that would effectively delay aspirin administration for everyone. So they agreed with our two-step consent proposal, but they want the complete consent process finished before the second dose is given at the ED. If the patient changes their mind and withdraws consent at that point, we have to drop them from the study and break the code on their packet to decide whether or not they still need aspirin. Dave doesn't think that'll happen very often."

"I hope not. So what's left to do?" Mary asked.

"Well, I've got to make these revisions to the consent document and include the interim analysis in the study protocol. Once I resubmit this to the IRB, they should let us know within about 2 weeks. Assuming they approve it, then I'll send a copy of their approval letter along with the required IRB forms to the community college. Once they approve it I'll send a summary of the study and a copy of both approval letters to the EMS advisory council."

"What if the community college wants something changed?" Mary asked.

"There's the rub. Then we have to go back to the hospital IRB and make sure that change is OK with them, too. Hopefully there won't be any issues that the two boards can't agree on. Keep your fingers crossed."

It took almost 3 weeks before Tom heard back from the hospital IRB. He was beginning to get nervous. He was relieved when he received a letter from the IRB in a standard, letter-sized envelope. He had already learned that the hospital returned the entire IRB packet whenever they requested revisions, so a regular letter-sized envelope meant it was either an approval letter or an outright rejection. Since the revisions had been pretty simple, he didn't figure it would be the latter. He pulled a pair of bandage scissors out of his pocket and snipped off one corner of the envelope. After putting the scissors back in his pocket, he stuck his little finger through the hole in the envelope and then slid it along the fold of the flap like a letter opener. The first words after "Dear Sir" were "Congratulations, your study. . . ." He smiled.

Tom was ready for this. He made three photocopies of the letter, then attached the first copy to the package of IRB forms for Katie's community college and placed the collection of forms in the large manila envelope that he already had addressed. He then took the envelope and the remaining copies of the letter into the station office. He put the envelope in the outgoing mailbox, and he put one of the copies of the approval letter in Mary's box. On the last copy of the letter, he took a thick red magic marker and wrote in large letters *FYI*. He put that copy in Timmy's box.

The community college IRB acted quickly, responding to the proposal in only 2 weeks. As expected, the board approved the study. More importantly, it didn't request any revisions to the protocol. The only concern expressed was about security of the data, but instead of requiring a formal revision to the protocol, the IRB chairman had simply expressed this concern in the approval letter. "The investigator must ensure that all data forms and other documents that might identify or be linked to specific patients must be kept in a secure location that only the investigator or coinvestigators have access to."

Tom knew that addressing the confidentiality issue wouldn't be a problem, but he decided to cover his bases. In the summary that he sent to the EMS advisory board, he described how all of the data would be kept in a locked file cabinet that only he, Mary, and Dr. Walsh would be able to access. He also sent a copy of the community college letter and the advisory board packet to Dave. He added a handwritten note saying he didn't know if the hospital IRB would want to see the community college's comments, and asking if Dave would take care of that if it was necessary.

Mary, Tom, and Dave all attended the advisory board meeting that next Wednesday afternoon. The board asked a lot of questions, and for a while it seemed as if the study might not be approved. Mary and Tom were kind of nervous, but Dave just sat there with a slight grin on his face. Eventually, the board agreed to support the study, noting that both a hospital and college IRB had already reviewed and approved the protocol, and that the board members were not making any judgment about the quality of the study design or the medical implications of the intervention.

"You have to be responsible for the medical implications of this," the chairman had said, wagging his finger at Dave.

"Yes sir," Dave responded flatly. He had been medical director for 7 years now, and he had learned this game well. The board members reveled in their opportunity to exercise—or at least threaten to exercise—some control over him, but in fact they never actually went against his advice. As long as he let them put on a little show of authority, they would always come around and approve his requests. Only once had he needed to assert his power as medical director, saying, "If any of you think you're qualified to make medical decisions, maybe you should go ask the medical board for a license. Until you get one, though, I'm going to make these decisions." It had worked, but it had strained his relationship with the board for quite some time. Now, older and wiser, he just sat back and smiled, knowing that eventually they'd defer to his judgment.

"Finally," Tom said as they left the meeting, "we've got approval from everybody. Do you realize it's been more than 4 months since we first started talking about this?"

"I know," Mary said, "and we've still got a long way to go."

Dave, walking between them, put one hand on each of their shoulders. "Hang in there. You're closer than you have been."

Mary smiled. "Thanks for all your help with this."

Tom stepped away, pulling his shoulder free from Dave's hand.

Chapter 10

Getting Colleagues on Board

It is a very rare research project that succeeds as a "one-man show." In each step of every study, the investigator is going to need the help of other people. In some instances, the researcher will need the expertise of others in order to design and implement the study. For example, reference librarians will help with the literature review and statisticians will help with the data analysis. In other instances, the researcher will need the support and cooperation of people who might not be actively involved in the research process, but who none the less can control or influence a study. A system medical director would have to approve of any change to patient care protocols. The institutional review board must agree that the study is ethical. Also, whoever is funding the study—whether it's a grant agency giving money or simply the EMS system approving the use of work time and departmental resources—will have to approve the study design.

While reference librarians and statisticians and medical directors and IRBs are nearly ubiquitous for EMS studies, the number and types of other people with whom the investigator will have to work will vary for each research project. If a study involves documenting dispatch and response time information, the researcher will have to work with the dispatch center director. If a study requires data abstraction from hospital records, the researcher will have to work with the medical records administrator. If clinical data need to be collected in the emergency department, the investigator will need to work with all of the physicians and/or nurses in that department. If a study, or its results, could have a profound social or political impact in a community, the researcher will need to work with government leaders. A successful researcher must be able to effectively communicate and interact with people who might have many different roles, priorities, and perspectives.

Of all the people with whom an EMS researcher must work, perhaps most important are his or her fellow EMS professionals. This is true for clinical, systems, and educational research. Without the support and assistance of colleagues, most researchers would be doomed to failure. Even in cases in which this support seems unnecessary—perhaps a search of computerized records or a retrospective review of call reports—the investigator will find, in fact, that involving colleagues in the process can be crucial.

THE IMPORTANCE OF COLLEAGUES
IN THE RESEARCH PROCESS

There are many reasons for involving other EMS professionals in the research process. First and foremost, in many studies they will be the people on whom the investigator will depend to conduct the data collection. Any study that will require field implementation of a protocol, or just field data collection, will require the participation of the EMS providers who work in the streets.

Organizationally, it might be possible for an EMS researcher to assign data collection responsibilities to field providers and to expect them to do so without question. In reality, this rarely works. There are at least two shortcomings to this approach. "Because I said so" is never a convincing reason for anyone to do anything. Children never buy that reasoning from their parents, and an investigator's colleagues won't buy it either. While they would probably do what was required of them in such circumstances, they wouldn't be committed to the project and they wouldn't go out of their way to ensure its success. Research protocols require attention to detail and constant evaluation to guarantee that the process is going as planned. An investigator needs the people at the heart of the project—in this case, other EMS providers—to have a stake in the study's success and to actively pursue the study question.

The second shortcoming to simply assigning research responsibilities is that the investigator misses out on the unique contributions that colleagues can make to the research process. There might be a better way to implement the study, to design the data collection form, to interact with patients, to measure response intervals, to structure a survey, or to do any number of things associated with a study. Having outside input from people who know the realities of the environment but who are not personally involved in the coordination of a study can be extremely helpful. Much in the same way as it is difficult for a writer to proofread his or her own work, it is often difficult for a researcher to critically and objectively evaluate his or her own study design. Bringing colleagues in from the very beginning and including them in each step of the research process will contribute to the success of the entire research project, not just to data collection.

The researcher must decide the extent to which these other individuals will participate in each step of the process. While "research by committee" is rarely successful, it is still important to be as inclusive as possible. The researcher can make it clear that, while everyone's advice is appreciated, the researcher alone must make any final decisions about the study. It is not a democratic process. At the same time, the researcher must be realistic about the importance of considering the advice of colleagues. While the investigator is the ultimate decision maker, a decision to disregard the advice of the IRB chairman might mean a quick end to the research project. Or, while it might be easier and cheaper to not revise a data collection form, failure to make the revisions might make data collection so cumbersome for field providers that they refuse to complete the forms. The investigator is in charge, but he or she must maintain a good working relationship with all of the other interested parties.

ROLES FOR COLLEAGUES IN THE RESEARCH PROCESS

Colleagues may be involved in each of the various steps of the research process. Some co-workers may be involved in only one step or only a few steps. Others may be involved in almost every step.

It might seem that the research topic would be decided long before an investigator would approach his or her colleagues, but this is not necessarily so. As discussed in Chapter 3, colleagues can be a tremendous source of ideas. Field providers, supervisors, administrators, students, teachers, physicians, patients, and community leaders can all be good sources for research topics. Pursuing studies that were inspired by colleagues gives the investigator a leg up on the process: Whoever inspired the project may already be committed to the study's success. They clearly have a stake in answering the question, and thus an interest in supporting the process. Also, those other colleagues who have ideas of their own will be more likely to support ongoing research projects knowing that eventually one of their ideas may become a study.

In conducting the literature search, the investigator may employ the assistance of a professional librarian; this is discussed in detail in Chapter 4. There are other colleagues who can also be helpful in this process. Many EMS professionals read extensively, and they might have come across helpful articles that may not be identified in the literature search. If a field provider knows that a researcher is exploring an intervention for asthma, for example, he or she might photocopy a local newspaper article about the high incidence of asthma in a given community and pass that along to the investigator. A traditional literature search would not find that article. Or, if a study is exploring EMS system design, someone who just happens to be taking a class in public administration might come across some useful information in the class textbook. Or, if a researcher is studying education of air medical services personnel, a colleague—perhaps the medical director—might bring back a copy of a position paper that was adopted by a professional organization at its most recent meeting. If a researcher's colleagues know about and are supportive of a project, they can be incredibly helpful in this step of the process.

As with identifying the topic and finding the relevant literature, colleagues can also play an important role in defining the research question and hypothesis. This can be particularly important in ensuring that the question being asked is the right question. If an investigator wants to study a new drug, should that drug be compared to a placebo—effectively, to nothing—or should it be compared to another drug that is currently used for the same condition? Those are two different questions, and colleagues can help to determine which is the better question. Or, if a researcher is examining response times in an EMS system, his or her colleagues can help to define response time. Is it the time from when the call is received at the dispatch center until the paramedic is at the patient's side, or is it some other interval? In an educational study, fellow EMS instructors might help to sort through whether an examination of two different teaching techniques should compare written test results or observed behavior during actual patient care. In almost every situation, what seems at first to be a clear and simple question can be further refined and made more precise by involving others in the process.

Colleagues can be helpful in determining the type of study as well. If the researcher is planning a retrospective chart review, someone who is familiar with the system's records can give the investigator an idea of how complete those records are, how easy they are to obtain, and how often they can be located. Having that information might change the researcher's mind about how best to approach the study. A researcher who is not actively involved in the field might propose a prospective study that is scientifically sound, but not practical in a particular EMS system. Field providers in that system might be able to identify this problem and the researcher could then revise the study appropriately.

An investigator's co-workers can be most helpful in developing the methods for a study. Because the study protocol must be specific and precise, the input of those people who will actually be implementing the protocol is crucial. They know exactly how things occur in the real world. People who are a little removed from the design process can identify simple things that might be overlooked by the researcher.

Perhaps a researcher is studying chest pain patients and specifies that a particular procedure will be conducted after an IV of normal saline is established. The investigator's colleagues might point out that most chest pain patients in the system get a saline lock, not an IV. The researcher can revise the protocol as necessary. It may seem trivial, but the strength of any research project is determined, at least in part, by the specificity of the study protocol.

In a study comparing test scores from two different paramedic education programs, the course instructors might point out that the tests are typically administered at the beginning of the 3-hour night classes, but in the middle of the 6-hour day classes. The researcher would have to worry that any difference in the test scores might be a result of the timing of the test administration, not a result of differences in the two programs. Having identified this issue, the investigator can specify that the test should be administered at a certain point during each class. These are just a few examples of small details that might not be apparent to an investigator. There are many others that might be revealed by consulting other EMS providers, administrators, physicians, local government leaders, or even patients.

Most of the help in performing the power calculation will come from a statistician, but other colleagues might contribute to this process as well. Since the investigator must make an estimate of the study results, he or she must have a good understanding of the current environment and of the potential impact of the study intervention. Consulting with co-workers can help with this. For example, the researcher might believe that approximately 10 percent of an agency's calls involve true life-threatening emergencies. Field providers, however, may estimate that life-threatening calls comprise closer to 20 percent of the call volume. The system medical director might estimate that only 5 percent of the calls are for life-threatening events. The researcher will have to reconcile all of these different perspectives in order to get an accurate estimate of current circumstances and the potential impact of any study intervention. While the differing opinions might at first be a source of confusion, having considered all of them will result in a better final estimate. Had the researcher based the power calculation on only his or her preconceived estimate, the likelihood is that the power calculation would have been inaccurate.

Success in obtaining IRB approval will depend in large part on interactions with the IRB administrator and, if necessary, actual members of the IRB. However, working closely with one's colleagues and with other interested individuals can make this process much easier. An IRB is unlikely to approve implementation of a citywide research project if it is not supported by the mayor or the city council. The IRB is also unlikely to approve a study of paramedic students if the course instructors are not supportive of the study design. Working with affected people in advance and securing their support for the project will be a valuable asset in the IRB approval process.

Colleagues can also help the researcher anticipate and resolve the concerns of the IRB. Perhaps they have experience in the informed consent process and know what things the IRB expects in the consent documents. Or, the IRB may be known to have concerns about including children in field research. Colleagues who have previously worked through that issue can advise the investigator on what the IRB will require, or if it is best to exclude children from the study protocol. Particularly for researchers who have never worked through the IRB process before, having the assistance of someone with experience can be crucial.

One's colleagues can even be helpful in getting other colleagues on board. Almost every setting has people, by design or by default, who provide leadership for the other people in that environment. If a researcher can gain the support of a senior field paramedic, for example, that might have infinitely more influence among junior field staff than the support of the system administrator. If a project has the support of the system medical director, it will be much easier to gain acceptance and compliance among other emergency department physicians. Of course, involving those influential people in as many steps of the research process as is practical will help to ensure their support and will subsequently help with getting other colleagues committed to the project.

Having colleagues on board during the pilot study is as critical as having them on board for the actual data collection. Their feedback will be critical to the ultimate success of the study. The pilot study is also an opportunity for the researcher to measure the level of commitment among his or her colleagues. If the pilot study demonstrates a lack of support, the investigator should do whatever is necessary to gain the cooperation of his or her co-workers. It's unrealistic to think that once the actual study begins, cooperation and compliance will increase. In fact, if one's colleagues are not on board by the time the pilot study is completed, it does not bode well for the actual study.

By the time the study is implemented and data collection begins, the researcher should have a good idea about the level of participation he or she can expect from colleagues. It is during this process that their cooperation can be most important, particularly if the researcher is relying upon colleagues to implement the study protocol and collect data. Even if a study requires little effort by these colleagues, their support can still be invaluable. By staying in close contact with everyone during this process, the researcher can identify and address difficulties and problems quickly, avoiding any critical impact on the study's success.

As with the performance of the power calculation, the investigator will work closely with a statistician during the analysis of the data. But, just as with the power calculation, colleagues can contribute to the analysis as well. The statistician will make mathematical analyses of the data and can report any statistical significance, but those who read the final research report will judge the clinical relevance of the findings. The investigator's colleagues can help sort through the practical relevance of the study's results. Field EMS providers can review the findings from the perspective of patient care, EMS instructors can review the findings from the perspective of EMS education, administrators can evaluate the findings from the perspective of systems design, and government leaders can evaluate the findings from the perspective of public policy. Each of these perspectives might suggest a different approach to data analysis, and the investigator, along with the statistician, will have to decide which ones are most appropriate. Also, having access to these different perspectives will be helpful when the researcher proceeds to the next step: reporting the results.

Writing the report for a research project is sometimes the hardest part of the entire process. It is not technically difficult or physically hard, but it is a time-consuming task that offers no immediate positive reinforcement. Because of this, the results of many research projects are never put into abstract or manuscript form and submitted for presentation and/or publication. Yet, sharing one's results with others in the profession is one of the most important components of the research process, and, as with all of the steps, it is one in which the assistance of colleagues should be welcomed. While "writing by committee" is almost impossible, an investigator's colleagues can still help in this process. The researcher can share drafts of the study abstract and study manuscript with co-workers, and solicit their input on the document(s). This has at least two positive effects: (1) it provides for a better finished product, and (2) it provides the researcher with some immediate feedback—some positive reinforcement. Colleagues can help to clarify portions of the report that might not be clear to people who were not involved in the study. As with reviewing the study question or the research protocol, having someone who can maintain some objectivity about the review process can be extremely helpful for an investigator.

ENTICING COLLEAGUES TO PARTICIPATE

For the researcher to recognize the importance of including colleagues in the research process is only half of the battle. The investigator must also impress that importance upon his or her co-workers. While some individuals are supportive of research endeavors simply for the sake of research, most people—in any profession—are not. To convince others of the importance of supporting research, the investigator will probably need to demonstrate what's in it for them. This isn't very altruistic, but it is realistic.

The first reason a researcher can offer his or her colleagues for supporting research *is* altruistic. Good research leads to better patient care. This is true for all types of studies, not just clinical studies. Educational studies that ultimately result in better training programs subsequently result in better paramedics, which eventually results in better patient care. Systems research that results in a better dispatch system eventually results in more appropriate response configurations, which in turn leads to better patient care. Even in the best systems with the best educational programs and the best paramedics and the best treatment protocols, there is always room for improvement.

There are at least two other reasons for supporting research that are somewhat (but not completely) altruistic. First, research is good for the profession. Working in a field that has been built almost entirely on anecdote does not lend itself to professional recognition. Those who have an interest in advancing the status of EMS professionals also have an interest in supporting research. Second, participating in the research process is an opportunity to learn. This is not only an opportunity to learn about research, but an opportunity to learn about whatever it is that is being studied. Someone who participates in a study about asthma patients—regardless of the extent of the participation—will undoubtedly learn something about asthma. Independent of the study's results, those colleagues who cooperate with the study will likely be better at their jobs once the study has concluded.

Of course there are many nonaltruistic reasons for supporting research, too. Sometimes, unfortunately, these are the more effective arguments for garnering the support of colleagues. Primarily, these reasons are associated with the prestige of participating in research.

If an investigator is trying to convince a system administrator to support a study, he or she might point out that the study could bring some recognition to the system. This would have public relations implications, recruitment and retention implications, or maybe even funding implications. Particularly if the study will result in some positive media exposure, the system could benefit greatly from this recognition.

Recognition can also be a selling point for individuals. In systems that value research, individuals who participate in or support research will likely be looked upon favorably by supervisors and administrators. Even within systems that do not overtly value research, though, there might be factors associated with recognition. Perhaps the medical director would be impressed by a field paramedic who cooperates in a research project. Maybe the program director at the community college gives preference to those who have participated in research when hiring part-time instructors.

If an investigator uses the promise of recognition to solicit support for a project, it's important for that researcher to ensure that the recognition occurs. If the system administrator approved the project expecting some positive press, the researcher might want to call the local newspaper and inform its staff of the project. The investigator might even distribute an official press release. If individuals are participating in the hopes of gaining recognition, the researcher might want to send a letter that lists the individuals and their contribution to the project to the system administrator, the medical director, or whomever else would be appropriate. Also, in any report on the research process or results, whether a preliminary presentation to colleagues or a full-fledged research presentation at a national meeting, the investigator should recognize the support of his or her co-workers.

One of the best enticements for helping with a research project can be an offer to include those who help as coauthors of any publication that results from the study. This can be a tricky area because most journals have very specific criteria regarding who does and does not qualify as an author. While it is important to recognize the efforts of those who collected data during the trial, conducting data collection as a part of one's patient care activities usually does not qualify one for authorship. On the other hand, a person who assisted in formulating the question, provided some advice on designing the study, aided in data collection, helped troubleshoot problems that arose during study implementation, and reviewed the manuscript for accuracy probably would qualify for authorship. If an investigator is going to offer a colleague a position on the paper, the researcher should specify in advance exactly what is expected of that colleague. It is also important to decide in advance the order of authorship, as there is some perceived status associated with different "positions" on a paper.

MAINTAINING ENTHUSIASM

In the early stages of a research project, the investigator's colleagues may in fact be very supportive. Whether for altruistic or other reasons, the researcher will probably find several individuals who are willing to participate in the study and cooperate with the investigator. In some cases, the colleagues may be so enthusiastic about a project that they actually push the researcher to move forward with the project. Everyone wants to get to the end answer as soon as possible. That enthusiasm, however, may fade very quickly.

When the research process starts to drag on, especially through the many months or even years that it can take to complete a clinical study, the investigator's colleagues will begin to lose interest. In fact, many investigators have trouble maintaining their own enthusiasm. The successful researcher must anticipate these doldrums and have a plan for sustaining some excitement about the project.

Regular progress reports are one way to keep people interested in a study. While the researcher does not want to conduct preliminary analyses and report the "results to date," he or she can let those involved in the study know how well things are going. A report on the number of patients enrolled so far, and the number that, for whatever reason, were not enrolled, can give colleagues an idea of how the data collection process is proceeding. It might also encourage them to be more diligent about enrolling patients. One way to share this information is to post a sign, similar to those used by the United Way or other community charity funds, showing the study goal and the progress toward that goal. Frequent updating of the sign provides positive reinforcement, and enables the colleagues to see how data collection is progressing. Also, since much of a research paper can be written in advance (specifically the introduction, methods, and some of the discussion) the researcher can begin working on the manuscript and share that progress with his or her colleagues as well.

Over the course of a long study, the investigator's colleagues will only endure so many progress reports. Another way to maintain enthusiasm is to simply invite people out to an informal social gathering—maybe dinner, maybe a bowling night.

Even if everyone pays his or her own way, simply getting together and having fun for the sake of the research project will help to maintain some level of excitement. It will also remind participants that the investigator recognizes the importance of their role in the project and appreciates what they're doing.

Another less respected but perhaps more successful way to maintain enthusiasm is through bribery. (*Bribery* may be too strong a term, but the idea is the same.) Perhaps some study funds can be used to pay for the dinner or bowling night. Likewise, pizza parties for the shifts that enroll the most patients each month not only promote data collection, but can even generate some camaraderie among system personnel. Having colleagues put their names on the data forms they submit and having a drawing for a "free day off" can be a successful enticement too. The investigator might have to agree to work that shift in place of the winner, but if working one extra 12-hour shift gets 15 more people to each enroll three or four more patients, it will be well worth it.

Some researchers are reluctant to use bribery, arguing that EMS providers should support research as a part of their professional activities. While most researchers would agree with that in principle, the reality is that all of us appreciate being rewarded for making extra effort. However, the investigator should be cautious about rewards. A few pizzas or an extra day off rarely present major ethical dilemmas, but any enticement for patient enrollment or data collection should be discussed with the IRB and funding agencies. It's important to make sure someone doesn't enroll ineligible patients simply to get a chance at some prize.

PRACTICE WHAT YOU PREACH

One final thing should be considered in the process of getting colleagues on board. An investigator who solicits the assistance of his or her co-workers for a study, but then is unwilling or unable when asked to reciprocate, will have a short research career. Indeed, someone who is planning a research project might be well advised to find and assist with somebody else's project first. It will establish the prospective investigator as a team player, give him or her an opportunity to learn more about the research process, and provide some bargaining power when he or she starts asking for help. It's a simple concept: "What goes around, comes around."

SUMMARY

No research project can be successful without the support and assistance of colleagues. Co-workers will play a role in every step of the research project, and the investigator must learn to make these interactions positive experiences. Involving colleagues in the research process has many benefits, the most important being that it results in a better study. As individual reasons for participating in a project vary, the researcher will likely need to use more than one approach for enticing and rewarding the participation of colleagues. Failing to engage one's colleagues in the process can be devastating to a project.

A Typical Experience
Part 8: Getting Colleagues on Board

"Man, this has been a horrible night," Tom said. "I can't wait to get home and crash."

"Arrggh. I hate you!" Mary put both of her hands to her head and squeezed as if it was going to explode. "I've got to stay over and meet with the B-shift people at Station I about the chest pain study."

"See, you should have done the IRB."

"You're right. I've still got four more shift-change meetings to go to, and if they're anything like the ones so far I think I'm going to have a stroke." She took a deep breath and then exhaled slowly through pursed lips. After a few seconds she said, "You don't reckon we're the only people who've ever wondered about this aspirin stuff, do you?"

"What do you mean 'we'? You're the one with the big plans for a promotion."

"Fine, Tom," Mary began angrily. She was about to tell him where he could go when she realized he was smirking. "Alright, you got me. I'm just tired of people acting like they don't care whether anything we do really matters. Actually, right now I'm just plain tired."

"Who's been giving you a hard time?" Tom asked, trying to be supportive.

"Nobody's saying they won't do it. It's just that there's always someone asking, 'Why do we need to do this? How long is it going to take? How many more forms are we going to have to fill out? Shouldn't we get paid extra for this?' Not a single person has said, 'Cool, what can I do to help?' "

"Not even Timmy?" Tom asked sarcastically.

"I haven't done Timmy's group yet. I meet with them next Thursday."

"Duh!" Tom was surprised Mary had dropped the ball on this. "You've got to get Timmy on board first! I thought that was why you had him in on all of those meetings in the beginning."

"No, I just had him there so he wouldn't work *against* us—not because I thought he'd do work *for* us."

Tom shook his head. "Here's your first lesson in management, Miss Supervisor-to-be. You may think Timmy is a jerk, I may *know* Timmy is a jerk, but most everyone else in this system thinks Timmy is pretty cool. Those who don't think he's cool are too afraid of him to admit it. Now, I'm not telling you that you can't do anything without Timmy's approval, but I *am* telling you that you'll get a lot farther a lot faster when you have him on your side."

Mary hung her head. "I can't redo all the meetings I've already done. I just can't."

"Maybe you won't have to. Let me see your phone."

Mary handed Tom her wireless phone. He held it in the palm of his right hand, punching in numbers with his thumb while keeping his left hand on the ambulance's steering wheel. He put the phone up to his ear, and after a few seconds said, "Hey, where are you?" After a few more seconds, "Yeah, it is early. Can you meet me and Mary at Station I in about an hour?" He listened for another moment, and then simply turned off the phone and passed it to Mary.

"Was that Timmy?" she asked. "Do you really think waking him up at 8 o'clock in the morning is going to help?" She sounded completely exasperated.

"Trust me."

Tom and Mary got to Station I at ten minutes before nine. Timmy was already there. To Mary's surprise, he was apparently bathed, clean shaven, and wearing his uniform. She gave Tom a puzzled look.

"He traded shifts with Mike today. Management lesson two: Keep track of the schedule."

Mary just sighed. "Thank you."

Mary finished her 15-minute presentation on the study, complete with PowerPoint slides and a two-page handout. She asked the group if they had any questions, and braced herself for a barrage of whining. She almost cringed when Timmy raised his hand.

"I don't really have a question. You came to me about this study a long time ago, and I've been trying to give you some helpful advice as it's come along."

Mary prepared for a long litany of problems with the study.

"I just want to say that it looks to me like this is pretty well thought out," Timmy continued. "I'm not saying it's perfect, but I think it's doable."

"Thanks, Timmy," Mary said, unsure of what had just happened.

"I know some of the other groups have had some questions, Mary. Instead of us asking all of the same questions, why don't you just go over those things with us?"

Timmy was being helpful. Mary was certain this was a sign of the apocalypse.

"Well, one big concern is how long the study will take. That will partly depend on how well people do at enrolling patients, but we're planning to collect data for a full year. That should give us plenty of subjects, even accounting for patients who refuse to participate, times that we forget to enroll them, lost data forms, and whatever else can go wrong."

Someone in the group asked, "When do you think the study will start?"

"We're hoping to start in 3 months. That seems like a long way off, but we have to do a small pilot trial first to make sure our protocol and all our data forms actually work the way we think they will."

Another voice asked, "How many data forms will there be?"

"That's been another one of the recurring questions," Mary said. "We're trying to keep it to a minimum. The plan right now is to have a card that you'll read to the patient to get consent, and then a one-page form where you'll write down information about the patient and the code number from the drug packet. The back of that form will have data for the ED to complete, and a space for the follow-up information, but you won't have to worry with either of those. To be honest, we'd really like your help with the forms. We're going to create them ourselves, but we'd like some of you to look at them and let us know if there's a way to make them better. Of course you'll use them during the pilot study too, so that'll give you two chances to let us know how to make the process more user-friendly."

The room was silent. Mary looked around for a raised hand, but there wasn't one.

"Another recurring question," she went on, deciding someone was probably thinking it even if they weren't asking it, "has been a sort of 'what's in it for me?' comment. We don't have any money to pay you, that's for sure. I don't know what it will be, and I can't make any promises, but I'm going to try to find a way to give some kind of reward to the shift that enrolls the most patients, or maybe throw a party for everyone at the end of the study. But don't hold me to that until I have more time to work it out."

"The other thing that's in it for you," Timmy interrupted, "is that you might actually learn something about taking care of chest pain patients. There's not one of you who hasn't forgotten to give aspirin at least once, and maybe now you can find out if that's a big deal or not. If it turns out that giving aspirin in the field doesn't make any difference, that'll be one less thing for us to fuss with when we have a patient with chest pain."

The room was still silent.

"So, if there aren't any other questions, I'm going to bed," Mary said, smiling. "Seriously, if you think of anything, don't hesitate to call me. We've still got a lot of work to do on this, and I can use all the help I can get."

"Thanks, Mary," Timmy said, more for the crew's benefit than for hers. "Let me know when the rest of your meetings are, and I'll go with you if you'd like."

"That'd be great." She couldn't believe what was happening. She looked over at Tom, who just smiled at her. She knew he had orchestrated this, but she had no idea how.

Mary felt pretty good on the drive home. Thinking more positively, she realized she'd already been successful in getting the support of a lot of colleagues. Tom had been with her from the beginning. Dave Walsh was on board. Katie was helping with the statistics. And Timmy, even though it wasn't working out exactly how she'd planned it, was turning out to be a team player, too. If he went with her to the remaining meetings, they'd probably all go as well as this one. Word would get back to all the other groups, too.

She knew enough to realize that this was only a small piece of getting the support of her colleagues. There was a long way to go in the study, and there would be plenty of opportunities in the future for her co-workers to lose interest. She'd have to keep them motivated through the yearlong process. She also still had to convince the ED staff to do their part. She figured Dave could help with that, since everyone in the department liked him. And she had to find some way to come through on her promise of a reward or a party. With nearly 150 full- and part-time field paramedics in the system, that was something she certainly wasn't going to be able to pay for out of her pocket.

She was afraid she'd toss and turn thinking about all of these things, but in fact she was sound asleep within minutes of climbing into bed. When she woke up 7 hours later, she hadn't moved the slightest bit from her original position, and she couldn't remember dreaming a single thing. Clearing her mind just long enough to make sure she wasn't supposed to be back at work that evening, she reached over to make sure the alarm clock was *not* set, and fell right back to sleep.

SECTION 5

CONDUCTING THE RESEARCH

Chapter 11
Conducting a Pilot Study

After deciding what to study, designing the study, and taking care of all of the interactions with other people, the researcher still has one more task before actually implementing the study and collecting data: conducting a pilot study. This step may be the most undervalued and most often omitted piece of any research project. In fact, it is at least as important as any other step in the process, if not more so. Conducting a pilot study ultimately results in a better research project. The pilot study allows the researcher to practice the implementation of the study, to identify weaknesses and problems in the study design and to make appropriate revisions to the research project before valuable time and resources have been wasted. It is, effectively, a dress rehearsal.

A pilot study incorporates every step of the research process, but many of those steps will have already been completed in the planning of the actual study. The topic will have been decided, the literature search completed, and the question and hypothesis formulated. The type of study will have been chosen, the methods developed, and a power calculation performed. Ethics approval will have been obtained, and the researcher will have already arranged for the assistance of colleagues.

The major thrust of the pilot study is to test the experimental protocol, the data collection process, and the planned analysis—steps that are yet to be completed. During the pilot study, subjects are enrolled and data are collected in the manner outlined by the study protocol. The primary difference between the pilot and actual study is that only a small number of subjects are enrolled. How many subjects are enrolled, or how long the pilot study goes on, depends on how long it takes to thoroughly test the experimental protocol. For a study that will involve reviewing 200 charts, the pilot might only include 15 or 20 charts. For a survey that will be distributed to thousands of local residents, the pilot study might include hundreds of people. It is up to the investigator to decide how much practice is needed before moving on to the actual study.

As the pilot study proceeds, the investigator can examine the process and determine what things, if any, about the study design are not working or not turning out as expected. Because this is only a pilot trial, these problems will not fatally affect the actual study. Indeed, the investigator wants to encounter as many problems and as many shortcomings as possible during the pilot study. By identifying these issues during a pilot study, the investigator can tweak the research protocol without corrupting the actual study.

The pilot study can identify shortcomings in any step of the study, including those that have already been completed and those that have yet to be instituted. Throughout the pilot study process, the researcher should be considering how the results of the pilot project might affect each of those steps.

The pilot study might demonstrate that an intervention technique, as described in the literature for emergency department patients, can't be performed in the pre-hospital environment. The researcher can use the findings of the pilot study to modify the technique in a way that makes it work. Or, if the researcher is using a medication dose recommended in the literature, but the number of side effects seems high, the researcher can go back to the literature for more information and consider reducing the dose or using a different medication.

If the pilot study suggests it will be extremely difficult to collect enough data to test a certain null hypothesis, for example one using "survival" as an outcome, the researcher may choose to revise the hypothesis and study "return of pulse" as an outcome. Or, if it appears that the effect of an intervention will be much larger than originally anticipated, the investigator might be able to revise the hypothesis and at the same time reduce the sample size required to test the hypothesis. Such changes are not inappropriate as long as they are made before the actual data collection process is started. Making such changes in a hypothesis after a study has been implemented and true data collection has started would be inappropriate. That's why the pilot study is essential.

The pilot study might show that the data needed cannot be obtained by a retrospective chart review, and the researcher could then revise the study to be prospective in nature. Or the pilot trial might illustrate that, while the data are available retrospectively, the researcher must abstract those data from the subjects' inpatient records because the EMS reports are frequently incomplete. The protocol would have to be revised to include review of the hospital record.

Any revision of the protocol would also require that the IRB review and approve those changes. Other IRB concerns that the pilot trial might demonstrate include problems with the consent process, with the ability of the investigator to maintain confidentiality, or with other ethical issues. By addressing these issues before the actual study begins, the researcher would be protecting both the integrity of the study and the privacy of the subjects.

One of the most likely areas in which a pilot trial might identify problems is with the cooperation of the investigator's colleagues in conducting the study. If field EMS providers don't complete the data collection forms during a pilot trial, there's no reason to believe they'll do it during the actual study. The researcher will have to find a way to encourage data collection. Listening to those providers is an important part of this process. During the pilot trial, the researcher should seek feedback and advice from those colleagues. It might turn out that something as simple as changing the layout of a data collection form or the sequence of the data collection process can make the implementation of the study protocol much more palatable. Whether they are paramedics, nurses, physicians, or even bench scientists, nothing will discourage the participation of colleagues like inconvenience. Making the research process as user-friendly as possible will go a long way toward the success of a project. The pilot study can be invaluable in streamlining the data collection process.

The data collected during the pilot project should also be subjected to the same statistical analysis as planned for the actual study. Through this process the researcher will be able to determine whether the tests that have been chosen are appropriate and/or practical. If the analysis was originally planned anticipating normally distributed data, but the pilot suggests that the data are skewed, the statistical tests might have to be changed. If the original plan was to report descriptive statistics as percentages, the pilot analysis might suggest that raw numbers would be more meaningful to the reader. The researcher should not use these trial analyses to draw conclusions about the study question; it's unlikely that any pilot study would have sufficient power for that. The pilot analysis is only intended to determine whether the analytical approach is sound.

As always, a change in any one step of the research process will probably affect other steps. If the pilot study suggests a change in the original question, that will likely result in a change in the methodology or the analysis. If the pilot study results in a change in the statistical analysis, the researcher will also have to reconsider the sample size calculation, and perhaps the manner in which data are recorded. Any change in the experimental protocol will also need to be reported to and reviewed by the IRB. All of the pieces of the research process are intertwined.

There are some negative points associated with doing a pilot trial. For example, if the study population is small—perhaps a specific paramedic class—then conducting the pilot trial might introduce some bias if the subjects for the pilot trial and the actual study are the same people. In a single-system clinical trial, paramedic behaviors could be biased in the same way. There are ways to limit these effects, the easiest being to ask another researcher from a different setting—perhaps a neighboring system—to conduct the pilot study. Unfortunately, that will leave open the possibility that issues about the setting will go undiscovered. The researcher will have to decide which is greater, the risk of introducing bias or the risk of not conducting the pilot in the actual study setting.

Another reason researchers often omit a pilot study is time. Conducting a pilot study almost always means that data collection for the actual study will be delayed. Often researchers are faced with deadlines. Deadlines might be imposed by funding agencies, or might be necessary because of an upcoming change in patient care protocols. Time can also be an issue if the researcher is hoping to finish the study in time to submit the results to a particular meeting. More often, though, issues about time are simply related to the anticipation and impatience of the researcher.

Whatever reasons (or excuses) one has for not doing a pilot study, they are rarely substantial enough to outweigh the risks of proceeding to data collection without doing one. Almost every study will encounter problems. The failure to identify those problems ahead of time and to rectify as many of them as possible is often catastrophic for research projects. Things that, when identified prospectively, are mild irritations and easy to fix can destroy a project when they arise unexpectedly. The amount of time, energy, and money spent on a pilot project is usually minuscule compared to the prospect of losing all of the work that went into, and the data produced by, a full-scale study that falls apart halfway through the process.

Some researchers who have a wealth of experience and a proven track record in a given topic area have enough knowledge about research in a particular realm that they are able to forgo a pilot trial. Those people are few and far between, and even they proceed with the understanding that they are taking some risks. Most experienced researchers understand the importance of a good pilot study, and would never proceed without doing one.

SUMMARY

The pilot trial is a test run of the study protocol. It gives the investigator a chance to examine each step of the research process: those already completed and those yet to come. By conducting a pilot trial, the researcher can identify problems with the study before implementing full-scale data collection. The pilot study is the last chance the investigator will have to go back and refine previous steps in the research process. While conducting a pilot trial can be challenging and can delay study implementation, the benefits of conducting a pilot study far outweigh the risks of not conducting one.

**A Typical Experience
Part 9: Conducting a Pilot Study**

This was the big day. It had been five-and-a-half months since Mary and Tom had first started talking about the study, and they were finally at the point where they could collect some data. Even though this was only the beginning of the pilot trial, both of them felt like it was a major step. The process had taken much longer than either of them had ever imagined, and neither of them had anticipated the amount of work it had taken just to get this far.

They had spent the month since Mary and Timmy finished the shift-change meetings designing the data forms, getting feedback from the other paramedics and the emergency department staff, revising the forms, and then retesting them. They had also spent a lot of time with the pharmacy at the hospital, working out exactly how the aspirin and placebo would be packaged, how the packets would be coded and tracked, and how the ambulance crews would restock from a supply kept in the emergency room. Dave had been a huge help with that, but it had still been complicated.

"How long do you think it will take before we find the first glitch?" Mary asked.

"About 12 minutes after the first chest pain call of the day." Tom was more matter-of-fact than pessimistic. "The only question I have is whether we'll be able to identify all of the glitches during the pilot trial."

They had decided to run the pilot trial for 2 months. It would push back implementation of the actual study a little longer than they had originally planned, but it would also give them around 600 chest pain encounters and it would probably give every paramedic at least one chance to run through the protocol.

Forty minutes later, when Sammy and Beth rolled into the ED with an elderly gentleman apparently having a heart attack, they were barely able to give report and move him to the hospital bed before Tom and Mary began hounding them about the study.

"It was fine," Sammy said, trying to calm them down. "He gave consent, no problem, and we gave him the four pills to chew. Here's your data form. The only real question was about home aspirin use. He takes Bufferin. That's aspirin, isn't it?"

"Yeah. Well, at least I think it is," Mary said, not as sure of herself as she wished she were.

"It might help if you could list the common aspirin brand names or aspirin-containing drugs somewhere on the data form," Sammy suggested, "just so we don't have to know what they all are."

"That's a great idea. Thanks!" Mary quickly looked over the data form. "This needs to stay with the patient so the nurses can get the rest of the data. I'll take care of this one, but just remember for the future, OK?"

"Sure, I know. I saw you two hovering here like vultures and knew you'd want to see it, otherwise I'd have left it in the room."

Mary and Tom hung around in the emergency department long enough to make sure the nurses completed the consent process and gave the patient the second course of pills. "You know, Mary," Tom said, "we can't stand around here for the next 2 months and watch every chest pain patient that comes in."

"No, but I want to stay as long as I can today. I want to see firsthand how the process is going. Plus, I think it just shows a level of commitment for me to be here while this is getting geared up."

"That makes sense, I guess. Do you want me to stay with you?" Tom was hoping she'd say no. He had a long list of chores to get done at home.

"Nah, go ahead and take off. I think Dave comes on at 3:00 this afternoon, so he and I can go over things if there are any major problems."

At the end of the 2 months, Tom and Mary were exhausted. They had both spent most of their days off collecting data sheets, reviewing consent documents, calling paramedics to talk about the process, and visiting the hospital to get feedback from the nurses, physicians, and chief pharmacist. For the last 2 weeks, they had been taking turns going to the medical records department and, if necessary, calling those patients who were enrolled early in the pilot study to do follow-up. They only had survival data on about 100 patients, but they thought that gave them a pretty good feel about how the process would go. So far, none of the patients who had gone home from the hospital had died, so they hadn't had to deal with a distraught spouse or child. They knew that would happen eventually during the study, and they weren't looking forward to it.

Mary had called another meeting with Tom, Timmy, and Dave to talk about the pilot study. They met in the same small meeting room at the EMS station.

"The bad news," she began, "is we only enrolled a little more than 300 patients. The good news is that, if we can maintain that rate, we can in fact get 1800 patients in a year's time. Still, I'd like to have some idea of why we're missing so many patients." She picked up a notepad and took out a pencil so she could take notes. "Timmy, what kind of feedback have you been getting from the other paramedics? They might be more honest with you than with Tom or me."

"I've been keeping a list." Despite his help with the shift-change meetings, Timmy had slowly been returning to his old, unlikable self. Tipping back in his chair with a yellow legal pad in his lap, he began reading. "There's the question about different aspirin brand names, but I understand you're already dealing with that. Another thing is that a lot of people were forgetting their laminated pocket cards with the consent statement. Some of them were just winging it, and some simply didn't enroll patients because they didn't have their card. It might help to put a couple of the cards in the drug boxes, or to tape them to the wall of the ambulance."

"Ooh," that bothered Dave. "I don't think the IRB would like the idea of people 'winging' the consent process. We've got to fix that."

"The only other thing I heard more than once was that there were some nurses, apparently per diem people, who didn't know about the study and didn't seem to know what to do with the consent forms, data forms, and the packets with the second dose of pills."

"I'll take care of that," Mary said. "I'll talk to the head nurse about setting up some additional informational meetings, and maybe we can do one specifically for the per diem nurses."

"Generally," Timmy continued, "I didn't hear many complaints about the process itself, but I'm still not sure anyone really believes this is a worthwhile study."

"Well, I really appreciate you working with us on this. It's a subtle thing, but I think you being involved gives the study credibility as much as anything does." Mary didn't like sucking up, but she could do it when she had to. They were too far into this process to let it fall apart now.

"Dave," she asked, "other than the uninformed nurses, how did things seem to work in the emergency department?"

"Not so bad. The hardest part is getting people to spend the time on the consent forms. I've been pushing them pretty hard on that. It does take about 10 minutes, so it is a pain. Still, we do consents for a lot of procedures, so I think this is more an issue of getting people to accept it as part of the chest pain process. The actual act of getting consent isn't that hard; we're just not used to having to do it when we take care of cardiac patients."

"So it'll get better?" Mary asked. "If we don't get the formal consent forms, we can't use the data."

"It'll get better. It won't be perfect, but it'll get better."

"OK," Mary turned her attention to Tom. "Tell me about the data forms, partner."

"We've gotten some suggestions on layout, adding the aspirin brands, and one person suggested using a heavier stock of paper so they don't get crumpled so easily. Those are easy changes, so I think we're fine there."

"Good." Mary stopped taking notes so she could give her own report. "I gave the 100 data forms with outcome data to Katie, along with some notes about the suggestions for changes, and she says there shouldn't be any problems with data entry or analysis. Of course, she looked over the forms when we were first developing them, so she kind of had a head start. She did suggest that we try to reemphasize to people that they should write legibly, but even she admits that's probably too much to hope for."

The four of them spent about 30 more minutes reviewing what needed to be done before they could start the study. They agreed that it would probably take at least 3 weeks to make the changes to the data forms and have them produced at the local printers. They also needed time to meet with the nurses, and Mary wanted to get to as many shift-change meetings as she could to give feedback about the pilot study and to assure everyone that their recommendations were being taken seriously.

"Can we shoot for September first?" Dave asked. "That gives us just under a month to get our ducks in a row."

They all looked back and forth at each other. No one wanted to say no, but they were all afraid to commit to yes.

After a few seconds of awkward silence, Mary broke the stalemate. "September first! Rain or shine."

Chapter 12

Implementing the Study and Collecting Data

When an investigator first envisions a research project, it is the process of data collection that usually comes to mind. Implementing a study and collecting data are what most people think of when they say "doing research." Yet, as has been demonstrated through the previous chapters, implementing the study and collecting data are only a small part of the overall research process.

Prior to beginning data collection, the researcher has chosen a research topic, searched the literature, developed a question, and formulated a hypothesis and null hypothesis. The investigator has determined the type of study to be conducted, developed the methods, and performed a power calculation to determine how many subjects are needed. The researcher has sought and received approval for the study from the internal review board, worked to gain the support of colleagues and co-workers, and implemented a pilot trial to work out any kinks in the proposed project.

Now, even while preparing to begin data collection, the researcher must keep in mind that there will still be much work to be done once this step is completed. The data will have to be analyzed and interpreted, and the results will have to be reported—first in abstract form, then in an oral or poster presentation, and finally in a manuscript.

PLANNING FOR THE WORKLOAD

The amount of work required to complete the data collection process will depend on the amount of data that needs to be collected and the estimated sample size, but it can also be a function of the study design and the source of the data. Anticipating the amount of effort that will be involved in gathering the data can help the researcher to plan this step.

Intuitively, it might seem that a retrospective study would require less work than a prospective study. The data have already been collected, and all that remains is for the investigator to abstract those data from wherever they are stored. In fact, retrospective studies often require considerably more work than prospective studies. The data must be located; the data must be accessed; the specific form or file containing the needed data must be identified; and then the data must be abstracted (copied) onto the study's data collection form.

The advantage of the retrospective design is that all of the data already exist, so the work—even though it is a lot of work—can be completed in less time than would be required to conduct a prospective study. That's not to say that all retrospective studies can be completed quickly. Sometimes simply determining where the needed data are located within a medical record can take a significant amount of time, and chart reviews never progress as quickly as one thinks they will.

If the study is done prospectively, the data can be immediately recorded on the study data form at the time of initial collection. Prospective data collection, however, is not necessarily easy either. Whether the project is a clinical, educational, or systems study, collecting data is an additional task. Even if the investigator arranges for colleagues to collect the data as they go about their routine activities, maintaining enthusiasm and ensuring protocol compliance take work.

In addition to the number of data points and the estimated sample size, the amount of work required for data collection is further affected by the study methodology. Asking 100 questions of 12 subjects during one-on-one interviews is more work than asking 100 questions of 12 subjects using a written survey, even though both collect a total of 1200 data points. When planning the data collection process and developing the study timeline, the researcher must take all of these issues into account. The investigator should also build some leeway into the timeline. Every study will be different, and the investigator will never know for certain how much time data collection will require.

WHO COLLECTS THE DATA?

There are many ways to accomplish data collection. The researcher may be able to perform all of the data collection him- or herself, or with the help of just a few colleagues. The investigator might also choose to employ individuals for the sole purpose of collecting data, or to depend on front-line personnel—clinicians, educators, or administrators—to collect the data.

If attention to detail is important, and the amount of data and the sample size are such that the investigator can reasonably do all of the work him- or herself, then he or she might choose to do that. The ability of an investigator—or a few co-investigators—to personally perform all of the data collection is primarily a function of volume and time. One person cannot reasonably review 10,000 patient charts; and while one person might be able to review 1,000 charts, two or three people could accomplish the task in significantly less time. It would also be difficult, although not impossible, for an individual researcher or a few co-investigators to enroll 1000 subjects for a prospective study—or at least to do so in any kind of timely manner. They might, however, be able to enroll 100 or 200 subjects. Again, it all depends on the study design, the number of subjects to be enrolled, and the amount and types of data that are needed.

There are enough advantages to performing one's own data collection that researchers should at least consider the possibility. Maintaining enthusiasm about one's own study should be easy (or at least easier than keeping other people interested), so the work might be completed sooner. The investigator might also be more careful during the data collection process, having a better understanding of how important small details are to the study's outcome. Also, when the investigator encounters an issue with the data that had not been anticipated, he or she can make an instantaneous decision about how to deal with that issue and be sure that the exact same approach will be taken if that specific issue comes up again.

There are also disadvantages to conducting one's own data collection. The amount of work required, and the time commitment necessary to complete that work, are only two issues. The investigator must also be wary of introducing bias into the study. Bias may be introduced when the investigator has to make a decision about some unanticipated issue, because he or she will not be blinded to how that issue is associated with other data points. Likewise, the investigator must be careful not to infer data—particularly missing data—from other information available in a chart. For example, if the pulse rate is supposed to be abstracted from the vital signs section of a patient record but the pulse was not recorded there, the researcher might be tempted to look at the ECG tracing and record the heart rate as the pulse. That could introduce bias, or it could simply be inaccurate.

In some cases, the investigator might recruit helpers for the specific task of data collection. These could be colleagues who agree to help with a retrospective chart review, students who agree to stand at a mall entrance and conduct interviews, or individuals who agree to help with data collection at a one-day mass CPR certification course. Whatever the circumstances, these helpers will have the specific and singular task of collecting data.

The greatest advantage of using such hired helpers—whether they're paid in cash, with meals, or with recognition—is the ability to collect greater amounts of data over shorter periods of time. There may also be less risk of bias, because such helpers rarely have a personal interest in the outcome of the trial.

The disadvantages of using hired helpers include their inability to make immediate decisions about unexpected problems with the data, and—more importantly—the impossibility of being sure that the different helpers are all making the same consistent judgments when unexpected problems are encountered. Also, because these hired helpers do not have a vested interest in the success of the study, they may not be motivated to maintain the same work ethic and attention to detail that an investigator would if doing the data collection alone. While compensation and rewards can be used to bolster motivation, they can also add significantly to the costs of a study.

In some studies, the only effective way to collect data is for the clinicians, teachers, or administrators on the front line to do it. This is frequently necessary in prospective trials, particularly those involving clinical practice or classroom interventions. These individuals will have to enroll the subjects, obtain consent, implement the study protocol, and begin the data collection process.

As with using hired helpers, one advantage of having these individuals collect the data is the ability to enroll more subjects in less time than any single investigator ever could. The data can be collected immediately, minimizing the risk of lost data or misinterpretation, and because—unlike some hired data collectors—these individuals are actually working in the field, they may have an individual interest in supporting the study. They might also be better able to make judgments about the data when unexpected problems arise.

There are disadvantages to this approach as well. While clinicians, educators, or administrators may have a desire to see a study succeed, they may not be motivated to do the data collection themselves. Data collection is an additional task that might be perceived as distracting from one's principal responsibility of patient care, teaching, or managing. Thus, failure to enroll subjects, failure to collect all of the needed data, and data collection errors can be common. The investigator will have to work hard to maintain motivation among these individuals, particularly if a study stretches over a long period of time. The researcher will also have to be alert to the possibility that such front-line people might have their own biases about the study question, and that those biases may find their way, either intentionally or unintentionally, into the data collection process.

THE DATA COLLECTION FORM

The investigator must make sure that all of the data collection forms developed for a study are user-friendly. This is largely self-serving: The investigator will be one of the users. Even if hired helpers or colleagues will be doing the bulk of the data collection, the researcher will have to use the forms when entering the data into a statistical analysis program, and, inevitably, the investigator *will* end up collecting at least some of the data.

Making the data collection forms user-friendly will also help with protocol compliance among the individuals who are collecting the data. Maintaining motivation can be difficult in the best of circumstances. If the data collection form makes the process more frustrating or time-consuming than it needs to be, that will only decrease the level of cooperation.

An investigator can do many relatively easy things to make data forms more useful. One is to ensure that forms are well laid out. For example, while shorter forms are generally better than longer ones, using a small font in order to squeeze six pages of data onto two sheets of paper is not a good idea. Using double line spacing and a font that is large enough to be easily read even under adverse conditions makes a tremendous difference. Lining up all of the data entry spaces so that the data collector doesn't have to move back and forth across the page is another helpful tip. Finally, the data points should be listed in the same order in which they'll be collected. There's nothing more frustrating than having a study data form that asks for pulse, then blood pressure, and then respiratory rate, while the chart from which they're being abstracted lists them in the order of respiratory rate, then blood pressure, and then pulse. It seems like another nitpicky detail, but it can make all the difference to the person collecting the data.

Another point is to keep the number of data forms to a minimum. The more forms the data collectors have to complete, especially if they have to complete different forms for different types of patients, the more likely it is that they won't comply with the data collection protocol. While some studies will require multiple forms, keeping these to a minimum will help to maintain motivation and compliance among the data collectors.

The types of data being collected—or, more correctly, the format of the data being collected—will also affect how easy the forms are to use. Fill-in-the-blanks data forms allow for more accurate recording of the desired information, but they also require more work on the part of the data collectors. This increases the risk of missing or omitted data. Another problem is that fill-in-the-blanks data forms can sometimes produce unexpected entries, such as a data collector writing *yes* in the blank for pulse instead of a number. There's also the risk of interpretation error, depending on how neatly the data collector writes, when it comes time to enter the data into a computer program.

Having the data collector circle or check the appropriate response for a data point is less work, and is effective when there are only a few possible responses for a specific data point. For example, checking or circling *male* or *female* is easier than writing out those words. However, circles and check boxes can affect the specificity of the data when they are used for other items. Recording the exact respiratory rate is more specific than circling *>24*, which could mean 26 or 46. Still, compliance with data collection may be better when check boxes and circles are used, and there might be fewer omissions.

Having the data collector or the subject draw pictures or mark a visual scale can provide very useful, very specific data. Unfortunately, these can be some of the hardest data to collect, and individual perceptions or interpretations can easily introduce bias. The directions for collecting such data elements must be specific, uniform, and followed consistently to ensure that data from all of the subjects are collected exactly the same way.

The researcher must weigh the advantages and disadvantages of each possible approach to data collection and determine which approach will be most appropriate for any given study. In all likelihood, the answer will vary for each data point within a study. However the form is laid out, and whatever formats are used for the data points, the data forms should be pretested during the pilot trial. The investigator, any hired helpers, colleagues, and anyone else who may collect the data should practice with the forms and give feedback about how to improve them. The statistician who will be conducting the analysis will want to review the forms to ensure that the data can be analyzed in the format in which they are being collected, and to check for the flow of data and the ease of data entry. The IRB may also want to review the data forms, although this will vary from study to study and from institution to institution. Whenever possible, changes suggested by any of these reviewers should be incorporated before implementation of the actual study.

Someone who has pilot-tested a form and suggested a simple change, and then finds that the change was never made, may be a difficult person to work with once the actual study begins.

GETTING STARTED AND KEEPING GOING

Once the data collectors have been identified and the data forms completed and pretested, the investigator can begin actual data collection. The researcher should set a start date, keeping in mind that there are issues outside of the study that might affect that date. It wouldn't make sense to start a study of near-drownings in Minnesota in January, or to start a study of paramedic students during spring break. Whatever the start date is, make sure that everyone—even people who might not be directly involved in the study—knows about it, and be sure all of the enrollers and data collectors have everything they'll need.

Once the study begins, the researcher will have to be available to the enrollers and data collectors to address any unforeseen problems. *There will be unforeseen problems.* The number of problems and the frequency of questions will decline as the study progresses, but the investigator will then have to turn his or her efforts to maintaining motivation. Enthusiasm for a study can wane quickly.

The job of maintaining motivation has many facets. The investigator, if acting as a data collector, must maintain his or her own enthusiasm for data collection. The researcher must also reinforce the motivation of others who are acting as data collectors. Finally, the researcher must maintain an overall level of enthusiasm for the entire research process.

Maintaining One's Own Motivation

Worrying about maintaining one's own motivation for data collection might seem silly. This is, after all, the investigator's own project, so enthusiasm should be automatic. It's important, however, to differentiate between enthusiasm for the project and enthusiasm for data collection. While a study might be interesting, exciting, and of true interest to the researcher, the process of data collection can be slow, monotonous, and boring. When the investigator is doing the bulk of the data collection by him- or herself, the process can also seem overwhelming.

Even if data collection has been well thought out and well planned, the reality of the amount of data generated by a study can be daunting. Imagine a researcher who goes to the medical records department planning to spend 2 hours sorting through the first 100 of a planned 1000 charts. Only 70 charts are there, and the average chart appears to be nearly 3 inches thick. Some are 6 to 8 inches thick. They're not in any particular order, which makes it difficult to figure out which charts are missing. To make matters worse, it ends up taking twice as long as the investigator had estimated to find the necessary portions of the chart. Two hours later, the researcher has abstracted data from only 47 of the 70 charts. It would be easy to consider giving up.

To maintain enthusiasm, the investigator should set a reasonable pace and plan appropriately. If 47 charts took 2 hours, then it will take about 40 more hours in medical records to finish the study. It's not practical to say, "OK, I'll spend all of next week here and just knock it out." About 2 or 3 hours of chart review is all anybody can stand to do at one sitting. It might be practical, however, to plan to spend 2 hours each day at medical records, and to plan to finish the study over the course of a month.

It's also important to set achievable goals and use them as milestones in the data collection process. Using the preceding example, a goal of 45 charts a day is realistic, and the researcher will feel a sense of accomplishment each day that he or she can get through at least that many charts. If the investigator can average 45 charts each day, the study will still be completed in 1 month's time. Having a secondary goal of completing at least 250 charts each week, and then, at the end of the second week, being able to announce to one's colleagues that the study is half over would also be an effective use of goal setting and milestones.

The investigator must take a long view and recognize that, although it will take a lot of work, the results of the study will be worthwhile. It might also help to remember that many studies take years to complete. In comparison, having to maintain enthusiasm for a few weeks or a few months should be easy.

Maintaining the Motivation of Others

Whatever difficulties with motivation and enthusiasm an investigator encounters in him- or herself will be even more severe among others involved in the data collection process. The researcher must remember that this is not their study, and they will not have the inherent interest possessed by the researcher. They will also find the process slow, monotonous, boring, and perhaps overwhelming.

Being available to respond to the frustrations of these people is essential. If the investigator is not available to provide support and positive reinforcement, other people will quickly lose interest in the data collection process. Positive reinforcement for data collectors can take many forms. Simply reemphasizing the importance of the study and using real-life examples of how the study might positively impact the profession can go a long way toward maintaining enthusiasm. It is also helpful to give frequent status reports on the study's progress. Knowing how much work has been done and how much remains can help the data collectors see the progression of the study, can instill a sense of accomplishment, and can help them anticipate the conclusion of the data collection process. This approach is not very different from the goal setting and milepost recognition approach that the researcher may use to maintain his or her own motivation.

One can also cater to the more basic needs of the data collectors. While some researchers discount this approach as bribery, the fact is that rewarding people for the work that they do is a fundamental component of how our society works.

Providing food—perhaps in the form of a pizza party or a group dinner at a local restaurant—as a reward for achieving a particular goal or reaching a specific milepost can help to maintain or rebuild enthusiasm for a study. Offering some other award for the individual who enrolls the most subjects with the least number of missing data points is another. Typically, the value of the reward shouldn't be so large as to encourage people to cheat, as that would adversely affect the data and thus defeat the purpose of offering the reward. Instead, it should be a token that is more a matter of recognition than of financial or personal gain. Indeed, recognition of any kind—announcing names at a staff meeting or publishing them in an agency newsletter—is an easy way to reward and maintain enthusiasm among data collectors.

Maintaining Enthusiasm for the Research Process

Separate from maintaining the motivation of the data collectors, whether the researcher is one of them or not, is the need to maintain motivation for the entire study process. One might think that the enthusiasm of the principal investigator for the study would be automatic. Sometimes it is, but other times it is easy to get distracted or lose interest. This is particularly true for studies that take an extended period of time to complete. As the study wears on, the researcher will be faced with new opportunities, new ideas, and the reality that he or she has other responsibilities. Few investigators are lucky enough to have research as their only responsibility.

It's important that a researcher begin a study with a clear understanding of the process and the amount of time required to complete a project. The investigator must also understand and anticipate that everything will not go as planned. There will be delays and setbacks. While these problems are never easy to deal with, knowing that they are coming will make them easier to tolerate. Understanding the realities of the research process can also help the investigator to ensure that he or she has adequate support, resources, and protected time to complete the tasks.

Even with good planning, a realistic understanding of the process, and the time and resources to both meet the needs of the study and fulfill other responsibilities, an investigator might experience some loss of motivation. When that happens, the researcher must turn to all of the approaches that are being used to maintain enthusiasm among others and apply them to him- or herself. Positive reinforcement, reviewing the study's importance, developing status reports, and implementing rewards are all proven techniques for maintaining motivation, and they can work as well for the investigator as they do for others.

MANAGING THE DATA

As the data are collected, the investigator will need to have some plan for how to deal with all of the data forms. If the investigator is the lone data collector, then, depending on the number of forms, they can all be kept together in one envelope, one file folder, or one box. If several different people are collecting data, or if data are being collected in more than one place, the researcher will need to establish a mechanism for getting all of the data to a central point.

If the researcher is using individuals specifically recruited to collect data, those people can deliver their completed data forms to the investigator on a regular basis—for example, every Tuesday. If field EMS providers are collecting data, perhaps the data forms can be collected in a drop box at each emergency department, fire station, or ambulance station. The researcher would then only have to retrieve the forms from the boxes. If surveys are being administered to several different paramedic classes in communities across the country, the instructors for those classes could mail all of the completed surveys back to the investigator.

However the investigator chooses to compile the data, it's important to stay on top of the process. The forms should be gathered on a regular basis, and the investigator should review all of the forms for problems or errors. It's much easier to correct problems when they are discovered quickly. While a data collector might be able to clarify whether a number on a form that was just completed yesterday is a 1 or a 7, it is less likely that this will be possible on a form that was completed 5 weeks ago.

The researcher should develop a system for compiling the data forms and keeping them organized. It might be helpful to number the forms as they come in and to store them in order. All of the forms should be stored together in one secure place. This might be as simple as placing them in a stack on the corner of a desk, in a file drawer, in a box, or in a large envelope. If the data forms include any subject identifiers, the IRB will probably require that the forms be kept in a locked file where they cannot be accessed by anyone other than the investigator or designated co-investigators.

Some researchers choose to begin entering the data into a database as the forms come in; others choose to wait and do all of the data entry after data collection is completed. The advantages of doing data entry as the forms come in are that the work is spread out over time and that the researcher can identify and troubleshoot problems during the data entry process. One huge disadvantage is that it is so difficult to resist the urge to perform preliminary analyses on the data along the way. While such analyses can be interesting and can even be used as feedback for maintaining enthusiasm, they're frequently misleading and always pose a risk of introducing bias. In the end, if the study design and power analysis required 1000 subjects for a meaningful study, then there's no good excuse for running the analysis with the 750 subjects enrolled so far. This is distinctly different from analysis by a data safety monitoring board, whose members are not involved in the study and which reviews the data to make sure the study is not causing harm.

After all the data are entered—whether entry is done as data come in or after all the data are compiled—the researcher should keep the raw data. Keypunching errors are common in data entry, and there will almost always be a need to go back to the raw data to correct such errors. Also, unless the IRB has specifically required that data be destroyed in order to protect subjects, the investigator should keep all of the raw data so that anyone who has questions or concerns about the data can review them for him- or herself. It's also a good idea—as with all computer files—to keep an up-to-date backup file of the data entered into the database.

CAVEATS

Up until this point in the research process, there has been much discussion about how earlier steps affect future steps and about how future steps might cause a researcher to go back and rethink previous steps. However, once the study design has been piloted, revised, and finalized, the investigator must then be committed to the methodology. It is not appropriate to change the study question, the hypothesis, or the methodology once data collection has begun. There may, however, be a need to fine-tune some of the process. Maybe the data should be compiled once a week instead of once a month, or perhaps the data collectors should be asked to enter *P* for the diastolic blood pressure when using palpation so it's clear the value wasn't simply omitted. But it is too late to make major changes in the study. The purpose of all of the previous work—all of those earlier steps—was to get to this point with a solid study methodology.

Even if all of those previous steps were completed perfectly, and even if the final methodology is as good as anyone could hope for, the data collection process will involve problems and new issues will arise. The researcher should expect these problems. There will be lost data, such as missing records or data forms carelessly left on a countertop instead of in the collection box. There will be bad data, such as someone writing *weak/rapid* for pulse instead of *120.* There will be peaks and valleys in the level of enthusiasm for the study, and that will translate into peaks and valleys in the number of subjects being enrolled. There will be something totally unforeseen, and it might be something that could drastically affect the study. All of these, however, are issues that the researcher will have to address without changing the study methodology. The investigator can track those issues and report them as limitations of the study, but the methodology for the study is set and the investigator should see it through.

SUMMARY

Data collection is the activity that is most associated with doing research, yet it is only a small piece of the process. All of the previous work is critical to reaching this point and to ensuring that data collection goes as smoothly as possible. And, even after data collection is completed, there are many more steps to go.

The investigator must plan for the workload associated with data collection, recognizing that many things will affect it. The type of study, the amount and kinds of data needed, who collects the data, the data collection forms, and the level of enthusiasm for the study will all affect the data collection process. The investigator must understand the influence of each of these and consider each of them when designing the study.

Maintaining enthusiasm among those involved in the study is one of the most important tasks for the researcher. There are many ways to maintain enthusiasm, and different approaches will be needed for different studies, for different phases within the same study, and for various individuals participating in any given study. The researcher might also have to work at maintaining his or her own enthusiasm.

Problems in the data collection process are to be expected, but a well-designed study will survive them. While the problems should be tracked and eventually reported as limitations to the study, once a project has reached the data collection phase, it's too late to make major changes in the research methodology.

A Typical Experience
Part 10: Implementing the Study and Collecting Data

It was September 1, nearly 9 months after Tom and Mary's original conversation about forgetting to give aspirin to chest pain patients. Even with so much work behind them, they were both aware of how much more was to come. For the next year they would have to be obsessed with keeping the study on track, and that was going to take a toll. In some ways, it already had. As much as they liked working together, Mary and Tom had asked to be reassigned to separate shifts so that one of them would always be off duty. They had agreed that they'd share responsibility for carrying a "study beeper" so that someone would always be available if there were any unforeseen complications that needed immediate attention. They had also agreed that whoever was carrying the beeper on Monday—every Monday—would be responsible for collecting all the data forms from the ED and taking them to the Station I office, where they were to be stored in a locked file cabinet. The person holding the beeper on Friday—every Friday—would be responsible for going to medical records and doing the patient follow-up. At least that part wouldn't start for another 6 weeks.

One good thing about being on separate shifts was that they'd be able to keep better track of how things were going and provide encouragement and positive reinforcement on a more consistent basis. To promote participation among the other paramedics, they had decided to hold a friendly competition between the three shifts. Mary, Tom, and Timmy would be the "cheerleaders" for their respective shifts. At the end of the study, whichever shift had enrolled the most patients would win a picnic/cookout. Dave had agreed to pay for up to $200 of it; the losing cheerleaders would have to chip in the rest.

As hard as this was going to be, Mary had a good feeling about it. Even though she would never have imagined all the work required in getting to this point, she was glad they had gone through the process in such a painstaking manner. As daunting as the next year might be, she felt prepared. Tom wasn't quite so confident.

The first 4 months of the study had gone along largely without a hitch. The few problems that had arisen had been simple and easily handled. One of the more difficult problems was when an ED nurse had noticed that all of a certain paramedic's patients were refusing to participate in the study. The nurse's curiosity was piqued, so he asked one of the patients: "It doesn't matter, I'm just curious, but was there a specific reason you didn't want to participate in the ambulance drug study?"

"I'm not taking any experimental drugs!" the patient barked.

Once this was reported to Tom, he was able to snoop around a little and finally got the paramedic's partner to tell on him. "He tells the patients, 'We're doing a study with some new experimental drug. You don't want to participate in that, do you?' There's no way anyone's going to agree to be in the study the way he presents it."

Mary and Tom decided it would be best for Dave to deal with this. Rather than fight what was sure to be a losing battle, they suggested that the paramedic simply be allowed not to enroll subjects. There would be no need for him to even mention the study to his patients. As much as they hated to lose the data, they certainly didn't need anyone giving patients the impression they were using experimental drugs in their system. Dave agreed and had a one-on-one meeting with the paramedic.

Now, at the 17-week mark, they were well into the patient follow-up data. This was proving more difficult than they had anticipated. Finding the needed information in the patients' charts wasn't so bad, and they still hadn't had to deal with a "my husband died last week, you insensitive boob" phone call. The problem was that medical records couldn't locate a large number of the charts. Usually these were the charts of patients who had been admitted to the hospital, and the charts were still up on the floor or in the office of the attending physician. Trying to keep track of which records they had gotten and which ones they were still waiting for was becoming a big problem. More importantly, the backlog was starting to take its toll on the Friday beeper person. Sometimes they'd go to medical records and find 16 charts from the previous week—the work they were supposed to do—and an additional 8 or 10 charts from 2 or 3 weeks prior. It was equally unfair to both of them, but that didn't make it any more palatable.

A bigger screwup had been that Mary had lost an entire week's worth of data forms. Even though she was on duty, she was holding the study beeper because Tom had to go to an out-of-town wedding. She had picked up the forms from the ED and put them in a file folder, and she'd put the file folder behind the driver's seat of her rig. She had intended to stop by Station I after her last call, but was so tired by the end of her shift that she had forgotten. By the time she remembered it 2 days later, the file folder was nowhere to be found. As irritated as she was with herself, she was glad it was her error and not someone else's.

Dave was mostly concerned about patient confidentiality. They could make up for the lost data by running the study for an extra week, but those data forms had patient information on them. He warned Mary, "I can keep this quiet for a few more days, but if you can't account for those forms I'm going to have to report this to the IRB. You don't want them hearing about this from some patient, or worse, some reporter, before they hear it from us."

With 8 months left to go in the study, Mary was starting to wonder if she had the stamina to get through it. The next shift, she found the data forms in her mailbox with a note from Timmy saying, "Found these in the ambulance the other day. Thought I'd let you sweat for a while." She didn't know if she was more relieved or angry. A mental image of Timmy toppling backward from his tipped-back chair and splattering his head on the kitchen floor gave her the answer. "Definitely more angry," she said to herself.

"So how does it look, Katie?" Mary was sitting in Katie's office as Katie dug through her filing cabinet looking for the folder with the aspirin study information. It had been 7 months since the study began, and they had finally passed the halfway point. Mary had given Katie all of the data forms they had so far so she could do the interim analysis for the IRB's data safety monitoring board.

"I don't want to give you too much specific information," Katie said, "but based on what you've got so far, I don't think the IRB will ask you to stop the study."

"I'm not sure how to interpret that," Mary said. "I guess that means there's no difference between the two groups?"

"Don't jump to conclusions. The only thing it means is that there's not an overwhelming difference one way or the other, at least not at this point. I can honestly say that—even having seen the data so far—I have no idea what your study's conclusion will be."

"You're being cagey, Katie."

"That's my job right now." She decided to change the subject. "How's data collection going? It seems to me you're a little behind schedule."

"Yeah, it's been tough. We go great guns for awhile, and then we have slumps. So, we go around and talk up the study and things go well for a month or two, and then they slump again. You know, it might help if I could give people a little inside information about how things are looking."

Katie laughed. "Nice try. It could hurt, too. What you can do is tell them they're past the halfway point, and that the interim analysis went well—meaning that the study protocol and data collection process are working the way they should. You have to make it clear to them that we don't have an answer yet."

"Any ideas on how to maintain a more consistent level of enthusiasm?"

"You're doing OK. You should be able to get a little peak in activity out of this interim report. Then you'll have two—maybe three—more cycles of slumps and reinvigoration, and then you'll be in the home stretch. Just hang in there."

At the 11-month mark they had data forms for 1273 chest pain patients. Tom and Mary were growing discouraged. In contrast, Timmy still maintained a smirking "see, I told you it couldn't be done" attitude.

Dave felt the study was going pretty well, all things considered. "Look, you've got a month left, and you only need about 300 more patients. That's less than 100 a week."

"Yeah," Mary said, "but lately we've only been averaging about 25 a week. At that rate, we need to go 3 more months." She was feeling like the last 18 months of work had all been wasted time.

"So if we can get that up to 50 a week, you can be done in 6 weeks. That's only 2 weeks longer than you initially planned."

"I can't really see that happening," Mary rubbed the heels of her hands against her eyes, "and I'm not sure how much people will complain if we decide to extend the study."

"What's the best week you've ever had?" Dave asked, trying to get Mary to cheer up.

"Back in the very beginning, we had a couple of weeks when we got around 70 patients. But that was when this was new and exciting. We're way past that point."

"OK, here's what we're going to do." Dave spoke as if he had simply taken charge. Mary didn't have the energy to object. "You tell everybody where things stand, and tell them that I still think this study is extremely important. I know it's probably impossible to get to 1600 patients before the end of next month, so I'm going to make a deal. I'll give them an extra 2 weeks—that's 6 weeks from now—to get to the 1600 patient point. That's 50 patients a week. They've beaten that number before, so I know they can do it. If they pull it off, then I'll pay for each shift to have a picnic—not just the winners of your contest."

"Dave, that's way too much." Mary appreciated the offer, but she couldn't expect that of him.

"I'll get some of the other docs to chip in. Don't worry about it."

"Are you sure?" She'd always known Dave was a great guy, but this was simply unbelievable.

"I'm sure," he said. "You *can* do this."

Chapter 13

Describing and Analyzing the Data

Mark Twain has been quoted as having said, "There are three kinds of lies: lies, damn lies, and statistics." In some ways, that may be true. Certainly, people have used statistical information in an effort to impress their beliefs upon others. A politician who received 50.7 percent of the votes in an election might say, "The majority of the people are satisfied with the job I am doing." In truth, the election results say nothing about the people's satisfaction. But that won't stop the politician from quoting the statistics. Indeed, many people believe statistics can be used to prove anything.

In reality, statistics can be a useful tool in preventing—or at least detecting—lies. If a reporter were savvy enough to ask the politician, "Exactly how many people voted for you?" he or she would learn exactly how big the "majority" is. If the reporter asks, "How many people didn't vote at all?" he or she has an even better picture of the truth. That is the beauty of statistics. When understood and used appropriately, they allow the accurate and precise communication of information. They also facilitate the identification of imprecise and inaccurate information.

This chapter provides a basic overview of descriptive and analytical statistics. None of these descriptions is complete enough to enable the researcher to actually conduct the test. The idea is to simply familiarize the new researcher with some of the common terminology that might be encountered during the research process. Ultimately, the researcher will need to work with a skilled statistician to determine the most appropriate way to report and analyze the data for any given study.

THE LANGUAGE OF MEASUREMENT

So how big is a majority? Fifty percent plus 1 is a common definition. Yet, when someone talks about a majority, a larger proportion is usually envisioned. *Most* and *few* are also descriptive terms that may not mean the same thing to everyone.

One of the roles of statistics is to provide standardized terminology for describing information. The statistical terms used to describe data always mean the same thing to everyone. This is very similar to the medical terminology used by physicians, nurses, and paramedics to ensure that everyone understands exactly what is being discussed. While a child might say, "I got punched in the belly," medical professionals would more likely say, "The child was punched in the right lower quadrant of the abdomen." The child's description is not inaccurate, but it is incomplete and nonspecific.

In actuality, the development of these jargons is not restricted to medicine and statistics. Lawyers, golfers, dancers, and divers all have developed jargons specific to their activities. Just as one must know what a two-line pass is to truly understand hockey, one must also know what the mean is in order to understand statistics. This chapter is designed to familiarize the EMS researcher with the language—the jargon—of statistics.

TYPES OF DATA

Data can generally be described as either quantitative or qualitative. The differentiation between quantitative and qualitative data was discussed briefly in earlier chapters. When describing and analyzing the data, however, a more thorough understanding is helpful.

Quantitative Data

Quantitative data are information that can be described in a purely numerical format. Quantitative data are also called *continuous data*. Heart rates are quantitative; they can be counted. Temperatures are quantitative; they can be measured. Minutes and miles are quantitative. Quantitative or continuous data—data that are measured numerically—can be further divided into two subgroups: interval and ratio data.

Interval data are numerical data that do not have an absolute zero. For example, while the temperature outside can be 0 degrees, that 0 doesn't mean there is no temperature. It can also be −12 degrees outside. The zero is not absolute. Another example would be the time it takes to brush one's teeth. No matter how fast someone is, it will always take some time. It can't possibly be done in zero time. Data that cannot have an absolute zero are called interval data.

Ratio data, on the other hand, are data that do have an absolute zero, or at least could have an absolute zero: For example, the number of cats owned by the workers in an office building, or the number of bicycles owned by each child in a neighborhood. It is conceivable that someone could own zero cats or zero bicycles. Data that can have an absolute zero are known as ratio data.

Qualitative Data

Qualitative data are information that can be described in some nonnumerical form. Qualitative data are sometimes called *categorical data*. The types of animals in a zoo are qualitative: mammals, amphibians, reptiles, and so forth. The types of salsa available at a taco stand are qualitative: mild, medium, and hot. People's eye colors are qualitative. Qualitative data, like quantitative data, can be further divided into two subgroups: nominal and ordinal data.

Nominal data are qualitative data that can be assigned to a descriptive group. The zoo animals are an example of nominal data. They could be classified as mammals, reptiles, fish, and amphibians. Another example of nominal data is American automobiles. They could be classified as Fords, GMs, and Chryslers. Although the descriptive groups used for nominal data differ, there is no relative value between the groups. A mammal is different from a reptile, but it is not more or less than a reptile. Although some car aficionados may disagree, Fords are not more or less than Chryslers, they are just different.

Ordinal data are categorical data that can be assigned to descriptive groups that do have some value relative to one another. Hot is more than warm, which is more than cool, which is more than cold. Likewise, excellent is more than good, which is more than bad, which is more than horrible. These are categorical data that have relative value. Notice, though, that the relative values of these groups cannot be described in a measurable, numerical manner. Hot is more than warm, but it isn't necessarily twice or three times as much as warm.

DESCRIPTIVE STATISTICS

One of the primary purposes of statistics is to enable accurate and precise communication. Statistics are most often used to describe data to others. These are called *descriptive statistics*. Using descriptive statistics ensures that others know exactly what was measured, how it was measured, and what was found.

As with all statistics, much of descriptive statistics revolves around the terminology—the language—of statistics. The differences between quantitative and qualitative data affect the types of descriptive statistics used. While this may start out as a source of confusion, it is quite helpful in the long run. Just by recognizing the words and phrases used to describe data, the EMS researcher can determine whether those data are (or at least should be) quantitative or qualitative. Conversely, if the data are known to be quantitative or qualitative, the researcher will know what kinds of descriptive statistics to expect.

DESCRIBING QUANTITATIVE DATA

The Mean

Probably the most common and most widely recognized descriptive statistic for continuous data is the mean. The mean is the mathematical average. To obtain the mean, all the measurements are added, and then the sum is divided by the number of measurements. The result is the mean.

In the following example, the mean speed of five cars observed on the local freeway is calculated. The speeds for each car are added together, and then that sum is divided by the number of cars.

Observation	Speed
Car 1	55 mph
Car 2	63 mph
Car 3	48 mph
Car 4	59 mph
Car 5	61 mph
Total	286 mph
Mean (286 ÷ 5)	57.2 mph

When someone says the average speed on the freeway is 57.2 mph, the EMS researcher recognizes that as the mean. The researcher understands that some cars are going faster and some cars are going slower. The mean does not say that most cars are going 57.2 mph; it does not say the majority of cars are going 57.2 mph. Indeed, it doesn't say that any car is actually going 57.2 mph. It is simply the average speed.

The Median

Because the mean doesn't provide much information about what each individual car is doing, sometimes the median is used to describe quantitative data. The median value is that value that has an equal number of observations above it and below it. It is dead center. In the preceding freeway example, the median speed would be 59 mph. Two cars are going faster; two cars are going slower.

Unfortunately, the median has the same shortcomings as the mean. Although it is the middle value, it doesn't convey any information about how fast all the other cars are going.

For continuous data, the median is most useful when there are a lot of observations with a few outliers that would mess up the mathematical mean. If two more cars were added to the highway observations discussed earlier, one going 58 mph and one going 130 mph, the mean would be 70.6 mph—about 18 mph greater than in the first example. The median, however, would stay 59 mph. Using the median in this way prevents outliers—in this case, the car going 130 mph—from misleading the reader. The median is even more useful in describing ordinal data, and it will be reviewed again in that section.

The Range

When someone reports the mean speed on the freeway—or the mean of anything else—it doesn't give the reader much idea about what is really happening at the level of each individual observation. If the mean age of a group of four people is 40, the group could include one 30-year-old, two 40-year-olds, and one 50-year-old. Or it could include one newborn, one 20-year-old, one 60-year-old, and one 80-year-old. Clearly, the two groups of people are quite different, but they have the same mean age.

One way to better describe the groups could be to define the range of ages. In the example just discussed, the first group has a mean age of 40, ranging from 30 to 50. The second group has a mean age of 40, ranging from 0 to 80. That gives the researcher a better idea of each group's composition and of the differences between the groups.

The Standard Deviation

The standard deviation is another measure of how the individual observations, or data points, spread out around the mean. Another way to think about the standard deviation is as the average difference between the actual observations and the mathematical mean. Although this is not precisely correct, it is a useful working definition.

The standard deviation is calculated by subtracting each individual data point from the mean, squaring each result, and adding all those squared differences together. Dividing that sum by the total number of observations minus 1 equals the *variance*. The square root of the variance is the standard deviation. It is a complicated calculation, and the math can be difficult, but the idea is to describe how much what is really going on differs from the mathematical average. Fortunately, many modern calculators and computer spreadsheet programs can perform this calculation.

Because of the way the standard deviation is calculated, 68 percent of the observations in any data set will be within 1 standard deviation of the mean. Ninety-five percent of the observations will be within 2 standard deviations of the mean. This helps the researcher or the research reader to get a better idea of how the individual observations are spread around the mean.

The standard deviation is most often reported as the mean plus or minus the standard deviation. In the first freeway example, the mean and standard deviation would be reported as 57.2 ± 5.9 mph. Now the researcher knows what the average speed is, and has an idea of how much what is really happening differs from the average: 68 percent of the cars should be traveling within 5.9 mph (1 standard deviation) of the mean, or between 51.3 and 63.1 mph. Ninety-five percent of the cars should be traveling within 11.8 mph (2 standard deviations) of the mean, or between 45.4 and 69.0 mph.

The standard deviation, like the range, helps describe how the individual data observations are spread around the mean. When someone reports a small standard deviation, it means that most of what is really happening is very close to the reported average. If the standard deviation is very large, it means that what is really happening differs a lot from the mean. The researcher must be careful, though. Whether a standard deviation is large or small depends on what is being measured. Is 10 minutes a big standard deviation for a time measurement? It depends. If whatever was measured had a mean of 20 minutes and a standard deviation of 10 minutes, that would seem to be a big standard deviation; 68 percent of the observations would be between 10 and 30 minutes, and 95 percent of the observations would be between 0 and 40 minutes. If the mean were 13 hours and the standard deviation were 10 minutes, that standard deviation would seem quite small; 68 percent of the observations would be within 10 minutes of 13 hours, and 95 percent of the observations would be within 20 minutes of 13 hours. One can see how the amount of variability in these two data sets is quite different.

DESCRIBING QUALITATIVE DATA

The Frequency

The frequency of an observation is simply the number of times that observation occurs. It can be reported as the raw number, or as the percentage (the proportion) of times that it happens. For example, a researcher examining the eye color of children in a day care center might find:

Observation	Eye Color
Child 1	Blue
Child 2	Brown
Child 3	Green
Child 4	Blue
Child 5	Blue

These findings can be reported in a frequency table as follows:

Eye Color	Number	Percent
Blue	3	60%
Green	1	20%
Brown	1	20%

The frequency of an observation is the primary way nominal data are described. Using the zoo concept from earlier in the chapter, one can imagine finding that 30 percent of the 200 animals in a zoo are mammals, 20 percent are reptiles, 20 percent are fish, 20 percent are amphibians, and 10 percent are insects. The frequency table would be:

Animal Type	Number	Percent
Mammals	60	30%
Reptiles	40	20%
Fish	40	20%
Amphibians	40	20%
Insects	20	10%

Notice how numbers can be used to describe the frequency, but the observations themselves are not numerical. There is no average animal.

The frequency is also the way yes/no data are reported. Yes and no are just categories. The number, or percentage, of times that someone answers yes to a survey question is the frequency of a yes observation.

The Median (Again)

For ordinal data, the median is the primary descriptor. Because each observation has a value (although it is a nonnumerical value) relative to the other observations, the middle value can be identified. For example, if patrons of a local restaurant were asked to rate the temperature of the coffee, the data might be:

Observation	Temperature
Patron 1	Cold
Patron 2	Hot
Patron 3	Cold
Patron 4	Warm
Patron 5	Hot

The frequency of each observation would be reported as:

Value	Number	Percent
Cold	2	40
Warm	1	20
Hot	2	40

But if all the data are arranged in order based on the rating, they look like this:

Observation	Temperature
Patron 1	Cold
Patron 3	Cold
Patron 4	Warm
Patron 2	Hot
Patron 5	Hot

The median rating—the one in the dead center of the list—is "warm." Notice that the ordinal data have relative value (hot vs. cold) but that the value cannot really be measured and has no absolute numerical meaning. If patrons at a bar were asked to rate the beer, the same categories could be used, the same frequencies could be observed, and the same median might be found. However, the perceived quality of beer with a median rating of warm would be very different from the perceived quality of coffee with the same median rating.

Another example of an appropriate use of the median could be to describe chest pain. EMTs often ask patients to rate their pain on a scale of 0 to 10. While the EMS researcher might initially think of that scale as quantitative data, it really isn't. EMTs usually tell the patients, "Ten is the worst pain you can imagine, and 0 is no pain at all." Those numbers, then, really represent categories. "Ten" is just another name for the category "worst pain you can imagine." It has no real numerical value. A chest pain rating of 5 is less than "the worst pain you can imagine" and more than "no pain at all," but it is not necessarily exactly one-half of the worst pain imaginable. In fact, the ratings assigned by chest pain patients vary greatly depending on their level of distress and personal pain threshold. A chest pain rating of 6 is more than 3, but it isn't necessarily twice as much pain.

If an EMS researcher conducted a chest pain study, the pain ratings might be:

Observation	Pain
Patient 1	2
Patient 2	4
Patient 3	9
Patient 4	8
Patient 5	6

It would be inappropriate to report a mean chest pain of 5.8, even though it is possible to calculate that mean. These are really qualitative data, and the mean is a descriptor for quantitative data. It would be appropriate, though, to report a median chest pain rating of 6. That is the center point. As many people have chest pain ratings above that as below it.

The Range (Again)

When reporting qualitative ordinal data, it is sometimes helpful to report the range of values. For the coffee/beer example, the range would be simply from cold to hot. In that example the range is not terribly useful. It can be more useful when there are more possible categories. In the chest pain example, the range of 2 to 9 provides a good description of how the ratings spread out around the median. In that example there is a lot of variability in the chest pain ratings. If the median chest pain rating for a group of patients were 6 and the range were 5 to 7, it would mean there was very little variability in the group's chest pain ratings.

The Mode

The mode is related to the frequency and is specifically used for qualitative data. The mode is the single most frequent observation of qualitative data. A listing of the shirt sizes worn by paramedics in a given EMS system might be:

Observation	Shirt Size
Paramedic 1	S
Paramedic 2	L
Paramedic 3	XL
Paramedic 4	M

Paramedic 5	S
Paramedic 6	S
Paramedic 7	L
Paramedic 8	M
Paramedic 9	L
Paramedic 10	S

The median shirt size is M. The range of shirt sizes is S to XL. The mode—the most frequent shirt size—is S. For the purchasing officer for this EMS agency, the mode is a very important statistic. It wouldn't be a good idea to order a large number of medium shirts just because that was the median size. Although the system will need to purchase shirts in all sizes, it will need more small shirts than any other size.

SUMMARIZING DESCRIPTIVE STATISTICS

This is the jargon of descriptive statistics. There are two types of data: quantitative and qualitative. Quantitative data have their own terminology. The mean is the average, and the standard deviation is, in effect, the average difference between any one observation and the mean. The median is the middle observation: the observation with an equal number of observations above it and below it. The range is the spread from the lowest observation to the highest observation.

Like quantitative data, qualitative data have their own terminology. The frequency is the number, or percentage, of times that an observation occurs. The median is the middle observation, and the range is the spread between the lowest and highest observations. The mode is the most frequent single observation.

Some of these concepts, and most of the math, can be challenging. But if the researcher is careful and takes time to think about exactly what is being described, he or she can learn to use descriptive statistics—statistical jargon—to communicate conceptual information about research data.

STATISTICAL TESTS

Beyond allowing the description of data using a common, uniform language, statistics also enable the comparison of groups, or sets, of data. Statistical tests can be used to determine whether any two or more sets of data differ from each other, and whether those differences are significant.

A word of warning is in order. Researchers—including EMS researchers—should not try to use the techniques employed by statisticians without fully understanding the principles and assumptions upon which these techniques are based. Although it is possible for the average researcher to conquer these principles, this book alone does not offer adequate preparation. While several statistical principles, methods, and tests will be reviewed, the EMS researcher should not try to use these without proper support and supervision. The purpose of this section is only to familiarize the new researcher with the types of tests used for different types of data.

BASIC TESTS FOR QUANTITATIVE DATA

During the process of designing the study and determining the sample size, the researcher will have to decide which statistical tests will be used to analyze the data. Which tests are used will depend primarily on what types of data are collected.

t-Test and Analysis of Variance (ANOVA)

Because both interval and ratio quantitative data are described in terms of their mean and standard deviation, usually they can both be analyzed using the same statistical tests. The two most common tests for comparing such data are the t-test and analysis of variance (ANOVA). A basic explanation of these tests is that they compare the means and standard deviations of two or more sets of data.

The t-test is used when comparing the means of two data sets. If a researcher looked at the effect of drug X and drug Y on respiratory rates, he or she might find that the patients who received drug X had a mean respiratory rate of 18 ± 4.2 and the patients who received drug Y had a mean respiratory rate of 19.5 ± 3.9. Is the difference between these two means statistically significant? Could the difference occur by chance alone?

The t-test determines how likely it is that one would find the same difference in means just by chance alone. If the difference would be found by chance alone 7 times out of 100, the P value would be reported as 0.07, and the results would not be considered statistically significant. If the difference would be found by chance alone only 3 percent of the time, the P value would be reported as 0.03 and the results would be considered statistically significant. (Although the t-test really measures the likelihood of finding a calculated t statistic by chance, conceptually it can be thought of as determining how likely it would be to find the difference between the two means by chance alone.)

The ANOVA is used when comparing the means of more than two groups. If a third group of patients had received a placebo, then the researcher would need to use an ANOVA to compare the mean respiratory rates of the three groups. The ANOVA determines how likely it would be to find the differences between the three means (or more than three means) simply by chance.

Again, the mathematical formulas for conducting these tests are complicated, and they are most often conducted using computers. The important issue for beginning researchers is to understand the language. The t-test is a test used to compare the means of two sets of continuous, or quantitative, data. The t-test can be used for either interval or ratio data. An ANOVA is used to compare the means of more than two sets of continuous data. Like the t-test, the ANOVA can be used for either interval or ratio data. Both tests report the likelihood of finding the differences between the means by chance alone.

Paired *t*-Test and Repeated-Measures ANOVA

In the drug X–vs.–drug Y study, there were two different groups of patients, and each patient received either drug X or drug Y. But what if every patient received both of the drugs, first drug X and then a week later drug Y? To find out if one of the drugs affects respiratory rate more than the other does, the researcher would want to measure the difference between each subject's respiratory rate after receiving drug X and his or her respiratory rate after receiving drug Y. There's a special test for measuring this mean difference called the paired *t*-test. The data for such a comparison might look like this:

Patient	RR after Drug X	RR after Drug Y
1	18	22
2	16	14
3	14	18
4	18	18
5	20	16

The paired *t*-test looks at the difference between the respiratory rates after drug X and after drug Y, and then calculates the mean difference and compares that mean difference to zero, or no difference. It asks, "Is the average difference between respiratory rates after drug X and drug Y significantly different from zero?" The paired *t*-test determines how likely it is that one would find the mean difference just by chance alone. If the difference could be found by chance alone more than 5 out of 100 times, then it's really the same (statistically speaking) as no difference.

There is also a special form of the analysis of variance that allows comparisons when the same patient is exposed to several interventions—or to the same intervention several different times. If a placebo had also been administered to all of the patients, and the respiratory rate were measured after that, the researcher would have had to compare the differences between all three sets of respiratory rates.

With such data, the researcher would want to know whether the mean respiratory rate after drug X differed from the rate after drug Y, if the rate after drug Y differed from the rate after the placebo, and if the rate after drug X differed from the rate after the placebo. There are three mean differences to look at, but all in the same patients. This type of analysis is known as *repeated-measures analysis of variance*.

Again, it isn't necessary for the EMS researcher to be able to conduct these tests or to understand their intricacies. The important thing is to understand that the paired *t*-test and repeated-measures ANOVA are the appropriate tests to use when analyzing the differences in the means of some variable that is measured more than once in the same subject.

BASIC TESTS FOR QUALITATIVE DATA

Because qualitative data are not measured numerically, they don't have a mean, so *t*-tests and ANOVAs cannot be used to compare data sets. The tests that can be used for qualitative data are called nonparametric tests. Which test is used depends upon the type of qualitative data being analyzed.

Chi-Square and Fisher's Exact Test

One of the easiest ways to report and compare the frequency of nominal data for two or more data sets is in a contingency table. For example, if the mortality data for a study examining the effect of two drugs on a terminal disease were reported, the data might be shown as follows:

	Drug A	Drug B
Lived	675 (74%)	730 (80%)
Died	238 (26%)	183 (20%)

That means 74 percent of the 913 patients who received drug A lived, and 80 percent of the 913 patients who received drug B lived. The chi-square test (χ^2) determines the likelihood of finding this difference in frequencies by chance alone. In other words, the chi-square test determines whether there is an association between the drug a patient received and whether that patient lived or died. It is important to know that the chi-square test cannot measure cause and effect, only association.

If the chi-square test determines that this distribution of frequencies would occur by chance alone 8 times out of every 100 studies ($P = 0.08$), then the conclusion is that there is no statistically significant association between the drug the patient received and survival. If, on the other hand, the test determines that this distribution would happen by chance alone only twice out of every 100 trials ($P = 0.02$), then the conclusion is that the association between survival and the drug administered is statistically significant.

It is important to recognize that the chi-square test formula uses the actual number of patients in each cell of the contingency table, not the percentage. Because of this, the study's sample size can affect the validity of the test. If a study has a small sample size, then a different test, the Fisher's exact test, is used to analyze a two-by-two contingency table. For example, a study with only 20 patients may result in the following table:

	Drug A	Drug B
Lived	7 (70%)	8 (80%)
Died	3 (30%)	2 (20%)

Although the percentages in each group are similar to those in the larger study, the statistical findings might be very different because the raw numbers are very small. It is unlikely that a chi-square test would be appropriate for these data. The Fisher's exact test is a special test for contingency tables with small sample sizes. Like the chi-square test, the Fisher's exact test determines the likelihood of finding this difference in frequencies by chance alone.

The Fisher's exact test makes an adjustment for small sample sizes as well as for small frequencies within a large sample. The Fisher's exact test is appropriate whenever the expected value for any cell in the contingency table is less than 5. (The expected value is calculated as a part of both the chi-square test and the Fisher's exact test.) Often, the Fisher's exact test is used to look at small subsets of a larger sample that has already been analyzed using the chi-square test or some other statistical test.

The Kappa Statistic

Another way to examine data in a contingency table is to check the agreement between two data sets. What if researchers wanted to determine if paramedics could accurately read 12-lead electrocardiograms? Paramedics' electrocardiogram interpretations might be compared to cardiologists' electrocardiogram interpretations. For any 100 ECGs, the data might be:

	Cardiologist Interpretation	
Paramedic Interpretation	*Normal*	*Abnormal*
Normal	68	12
Abnormal	7	13

The cardiologists and the paramedics agreed on 81 of the 100 ECGs: 68 normal ECGs and 13 abnormal ECGs. Is this good agreement? It is not 100 percent agreement, but, given the role of chance in statistics, 100 percent agreement will probably never happen. So what level of agreement is good enough?

Even if the paramedics just guessed at the ECG interpretation, without having any idea about how to read an ECG, they could have guessed right at least some of the time just by chance alone. The kappa (κ) statistic is a measurement of how much agreement exists beyond that which would occur by chance alone. Unlike other statistical tests, though, kappa does not report a P value. Instead, a kappa statistic is reported as a value between 0 and 1, with 0 being no agreement beyond chance alone and 1 being absolutely perfect agreement. A kappa of 0.6 or greater is usually used to signify substantial agreement between data sets.

Wilcoxon Rank Sum Test

The chi-square test, the Fisher's exact test, and the kappa statistic are all tests used exclusively for nominal data that can be placed into a contingency table. A completely different cadre of tests is used for analyzing ordinal data. The Wilcoxon rank sum test is one of those tests.

The Wilcoxon rank sum test compares the median ranking of two sets of data. In concept, it is similar to using the *t*-test to compare the means of two groups of continuous data. The Wilcoxon rank sum test compares the rankings assigned to two groups of data, calculates the median and range of rankings, and determines how likely it is that the differences in those rankings would occur by chance alone.

If a researcher were comparing the temperature of the hot chocolate at two local restaurants and asked a half dozen customers to describe the product, the data might be:

Observation	Restaurant 1	Restaurant 2
Patron 1	Hot	Hot
Patron 2	Hot	Warm
Patron 3	Warm	Warm
Patron 4	Hot	Warm
Patron 5	Cool	Warm
Patron 6	Warm	Hot

Restaurant 1 has more "hot" rankings than restaurant 2, but it also has the only "cool" ranking. Is there really a difference in the rankings of the hot chocolate for restaurant 1 and restaurant 2? Restaurant 1's hot chocolate has a median ranking that is halfway between warm and hot, ranging from hot to cool. Restaurant 2 has a median ranking of warm, ranging from hot to warm. These rankings are different, and the Wilcoxon test determines how likely it is that one would find this difference in rankings by chance alone. If the Wilcoxon test produces a P value less than 0.05, the difference in rankings is considered statistically significant.

It is important to note that, in order to make the analysis of ratings easier, researchers frequently assign numerical values to ratings. In this example, 1 could be assigned to hot, 2 to warm, and 3 to cool. This is only done to help with data management and statistical calculations. The numbers have no true value and no specific value relative to each other. They are simply used because it is easier to write numbers than to write out words. It's just like when an EMS provider asks a chest pain patient to rate his or her pain on a scale of 0 to 10. These numerical values that are assigned to ordinal data are sometimes called *dummy variables*.

Wilcoxon Rank Sign Test

A special t-test is used to look at the mean differences between pairs of data. There is also a special test to look at the differences between the rankings of paired data. In a before-and-after study, for example, the Wilcoxon rank sign test would determine the difference in each subject's rankings before and after an intervention. The test would then determine the median change in ranking, and how likely it is that one would find this median change in ranking just by chance alone. Another way to think of this is: The Wilcoxon rank sign test determines whether the change in ranking is significantly different from zero, or no change.

Kruskal-Wallis Test

Just as the ANOVA is a special test for comparing data sets with more than two means, there is a special test for comparing data involving more than two medians or more than two sets of rankings. It is called the Kruskal-Wallis test. The Kruskal-Wallis test compares the median rankings of more than two groups of data. Like the

Wilcoxon rank sum test, the Kruskal-Wallis test determines how likely it is that the differences in the rankings would occur by chance alone.

One shortcoming of the Kruskal-Wallis test is that it can only determine that the median rankings for the three or more data sets are different. It cannot determine which of the sets differ from each other, or by how much. There are other special tests, most notably Dunn's procedure, for making those determinations.

CONFIDENCE INTERVALS

Because of the influence of chance, the findings of any single study are unlikely to be exact. They are only an estimate based on the study population. Confidence intervals help to account for the error that can occur in any single study. They are a statistical calculation that can bridge descriptive and analytical statistics, and they can be used for quantitative and qualitative data. They can be quite useful in examining data.

Suppose a study of 10 EMS systems finds that 17 percent of EMTs have back injuries. Does that mean that 17 percent of all EMTs nationwide have back injuries? Probably not. Is the actual proportion 18 percent? Or is it 15 percent? Confidence intervals cannot determine the actual rate of injury among all EMTs, but they can estimate a range within which that number is likely to fall.

A unique aspect of confidence intervals is that they can be calculated for many types of data. They can be calculated for a mean (continuous data), and they can be calculated for a percentage (frequency data). A confidence interval can be calculated around a kappa statistic, an odds ratio, or any number of other statistical constructs.

Typically researchers use what are known as *95 percent confidence intervals.* That means that there is a 95 percent chance that the true value for a given study finding will lie somewhere within the calculated range. Put another way, if the same study is conducted exactly the same way 100 times, in 95 percent of those studies the results will fall within the calculated range.

So, if a study reports a mean heart rate for golfers of 80, with a 95 percent confidence interval of 76 to 85, that means there's a 95 percent chance that the true mean heart rate of all golfers in the universe is somewhere between 76 and 85. If a study reports that 63 percent of stroke patients have one-sided weakness, with a 95 percent confidence interval of 54 percent to 75 percent, that means there's a 95 percent chance that the actual proportion of all stroke patients who have one-sided weakness is somewhere between 54 and 75 percent.

Researchers can use confidence intervals to help with comparing data sets by examining the overlap of the confidence intervals for two different groups. If the intervals overlap, then the groups are not statistically different. Consider two groups of patients who have had their diastolic blood pressure measured:

Group	Mean DBP	95 % Confidence Interval
A	87	78 to 96
B	83	74 to 92

Although the mean diastolic blood pressures differ, the 95 percent confidence intervals for the two groups overlap. So, the researcher can conclude that the groups are not statistically different with regards to diastolic blood pressure.

If the proportion of trauma patients who survive in a two-armed study is:

Arm	Survival	95% Confidence Interval
I	95%	94% to 96%
II	92%	91% to 93%

the researcher can conclude that survival is greater in arm I than in arm II; the 95 percent confidence intervals do not overlap.

When comparing the difference between data sets (when comparing paired data), the researcher can calculate a 95 percent confidence interval around that difference. If the 95 percent confidence interval for the difference overlaps zero (no difference), that means the difference between the groups is not statistically significant.

The use of confidence intervals is becoming more and more common, and many medical journals prefer to have confidence intervals reported instead of P values. But again, it is not necessary for the new researcher to master the math. The statistician can help with calculating these intervals and in determining the best way to report the results.

SUMMARY

Statistics are a way of communicating data using standardized terminology. There are different types of data, and the terminology used to describe data varies by the type of data. In addition to describing data, statistics are used to analyze the differences between sets of data. As with the descriptive terminology, the statistical tests used to analyze data differ depending on the type of data. In general, though, statistical tests provide a measurement of how often the differences between data sets would occur simply by chance alone. Usually, if the difference would occur by chance alone 5 or more times out of every 100 trials, that difference is not considered statistically significant.

This chapter has reviewed only a few of the statistical tests available for analyzing data. These are, however, some of the more common tests. Odds ratios, likelihood ratios, linear regression, logistic regression, correlation coefficients, and many other statistical procedures have not been discussed. Each of these tests has an appropriate use depending on the type of data being analyzed.

This overview of the statistical tests available for examining various types of data is only intended to give the EMS researcher a general understanding of the complexities involved in data analysis. None of these descriptions is complete enough to enable the researcher to actually conduct the test. Any one of these statistical techniques could be the subject of an entire textbook, or an entire college course. Hopefully, though, these explanations will give the researcher some idea of the tests that might be appropriate for certain types of data. Ultimately, the researcher will need to work with a skilled statistician to determine the most appropriate test for any given study, as well as to conduct the analysis.

The mathematical formulas and theories used to conduct all of these tests are quite complicated. The purpose of this chapter is not to teach the EMS researcher how to conduct these tests, but to familiarize the researcher with the types of tests that are appropriate for different types of data. When reading the published literature, and when planning a study, it is important to know which tests are proper and which tests are not.

The statistician plays an important role in every step of the research process. Even the most experienced researchers can make use of a statistician. There are many rules and assumptions associated with each statistical test. It is the statistician's job to understand these subtleties and to select the appropriate tests. Statisticians can be found at medical schools, universities, community colleges, and in local government.

The EMS researcher, or any researcher, must understand his or her own limitations when it comes to statistics. It is important to recognize when help is needed and not to be afraid to ask for it.

A Typical Experience
Part 11: Describing and Analyzing the Data

Mary looked around at the crowd gathered at Mill Creek Park. There were 47 paramedics on C-shift, and, with spouses, boyfriends, girlfriends, and children, there had to be at least 150 people at the picnic. She looked up at the banner dangling from the rafters of the shelter, suspended there by fraying lengths of twine. "1607" was painted on it in large red numerals. This was the third and last picnic, and that was probably a good thing. The paper banner was tattered and torn, and looked as if it were about to disintegrate.

"Dave, I can't believe you did all this. It must have cost a fortune." She hesitated for a moment, and then added awkwardly, "I'd hug you, but I'm afraid people would talk."

Dave grinned and shook his head with understanding. "It's alright, Mary. I was able to get some of the drug companies to make a significant contribution toward this. That's why all the cups and napkins have logos on them. Don't forget to load up on those ballpoint pens, too."

"I hope you didn't promise them we'd do a prehospital thrombolytic study." She was only half-faking exasperation.

"No promises at all. This is an unrestricted educational grant. So, educate me. How are the data looking?"

"I met with Katie last week. She's got everything broken down nicely."

Mary explained how Katie had prepared several tables summarizing the data. The first table compared the two groups of patients based on the characteristics the EMS providers had recorded: age, sex, duration of pain, and previous aspirin use. She told Dave that the two groups were not exactly the same, but that they were similar enough that the study results should be valid. There was only a 1-year difference in their average age, only a 6-minute difference in the average duration of symptoms, only a 2 percent difference in the proportions of males and females, and only a 1 percent difference in the frequency of home aspirin use.

"What about the survival data?" Dave asked. "That's the bottom line, right?"

"I don't know about that yet. I'm meeting with Katie next week to do the final analysis."

"Katie, I appreciate all you've done for us, and I really appreciate you letting me watch you work through this analysis. I know it would be easier and faster if I wasn't looking over your shoulder."

"That's OK, Mary." Katie pulled one of the metal and plastic chairs around to her side of the desk so Mary could see what she was doing. "I am a teacher, after all. This is fun for me."

"I hope so. Can you explain this table to me again? I mean, I can see that the numbers aren't very different, but what are all these tests mentioned in the footnotes?"

"Here," Katie said, holding the table between the two of them so they could both see it. "Things like age and time that you measure numerically are usually reported as the mean, or the average."

"I've got that."

"So this test, the *t*-test, is a statistical test that compares averages. I'm not sure you really want to know any more than that."

"You can't tell me how it works?" Mary asked, truly curious.

"Well, I can, but it's not very simple, and I don't think you really need to understand that. Think of it this way, how do you tell the difference between, say, Coke and Pepsi?"

Mary looked confused. "By reading the label on the bottle. How else?"

"Well, actually, I was thinking by taste, but it doesn't matter. The point is, you don't have to know all the intricacies of how your eyes work—or how your taste buds work—to know that you can use them to differentiate between Coke and Pepsi. Your tongue and eyes are tools. The *t*-test is a tool; it's a tool we use to compare means—or averages."

"I guess I can live with that. What about these, then?" she asked, pointing to the sex and aspirin use data.

"Ah," Katie said, holding her index finger up in the air. "Those are percentages, or frequencies. You can't use a *t*-test for those; they're different. Do you use your eyes to tell whether or not a swimming pool is heated?"

Mary shook her head, as much to indicate she was confused again as to say no. "I usually stick my toe in the water."

"That's right!" Katie was honestly excited by this. "It's a different type of information, a different type of data. So, you need a different test! We use a *t*-test for means, but we use a test called chi-square for frequencies—for percentages."

"I have no idea what Coke and Pepsi and pool water have to do with analyzing my aspirin study, Katie. Maybe I better go and just let you do this."

"No, no, no. You stay here. These are baby steps for you. I don't expect you to get it all right away. Just let it sink in. The important thing is, don't think of it as math—that's what gets most people in trouble."

"If you say so."

"I do. Now, what these tests say is that the differences between these groups—between the aspirin and the no-aspirin patients—are probably just a function of chance. Just by dumb luck, if you picked any two groups of 800 patients, they'd be a little bit different. These data say that your two groups probably aren't any more different than any other two groups of people would be."

"This part I think I get," Mary said, encouraged. "That's why they all have P values bigger than 0.05; that means the differences aren't very big."

"That's an OK way to think about it," Katie corrected, "but the statistical test doesn't really say much about the size of the difference, it just says the difference could have happened by chance alone. But you're right, you can interpret that as meaning the differences between the groups are minimal."

"So that's good, right? Now what about the survival stuff?" Mary was growing anxious about the results.

"Alright, look at this." Katie showed her another table. This one was a breakdown of the patients by their randomization. "It didn't work out exactly 50-50, but that's to be expected. You had 783 patients in the aspirin group, and 11 of them died. You had 824 patients in the no-aspirin group, and 24 of them died."

"Is that a big difference?" Mary asked.

"Well, you tell me," Katie said. "That's 1.4 percent vs. 2.9 percent."

Mary thought about it a few seconds. "I don't know. A 1.5 percent difference doesn't seem like much, but 2.9 percent is more than double 1.4 percent. I guess I really don't know."

"Let me get you to think about it differently," Katie said. "Remember when we did the power calculation? We estimated the no-aspirin mortality rate would be 3 percent, right?"

"Right, and we said we wanted to be able to show a statistical difference if the aspirin group death rate was 1 percent."

"That's right," Katie said.

"Oh," Mary was getting it now. "But we didn't find the exact numbers we were looking for, and the aspirin death rate is 1.4 percent, not 1 percent. Does that mean it's not significant?"

"Well, let's work on this a little more. In the no-aspirin group, if you treated 100 people, how many would die?"

Mary hated math questions. "Um . . . 2.9 people?"

Katie smiled, "Let's say three. Now, what if you took care of 200 people?"

"That's double, so six people would die."

"Right, now what about the aspirin group?" Katie liked teaching, and she particularly liked coaching students to figure things out on their own. "How many out of 200 aspirin patients would die?"

Mary picked up a pencil and a piece of scrap paper. "Let's see, 1.4 doubled is . . . 2.8 . . . so . . . about 3 out of 200 would die." A smile began to creep across her lips. "So 6 out of every 200 no-aspirin chest pain patients died, and only three out of every 200 patients who got aspirin died! I guess that is significant."

"Halfway there!" Katie said. "You believe the difference is big enough to be clinically relevant. That's good. Now we have to figure out how likely it is that the difference happened just by chance, just by dumb luck."

Katie launched a statistical analysis program on her computer, and punched in the numbers she had scribbled on her notepad. "There, using chi-square the P value is 0.038. So there you go. The statistical test says that there's less than a 4 percent chance that the difference happened just by chance alone!"

"So aspirin is good," Mary confirmed.

"Well, having aspirin in the chest pain protocol is good. Remember, you had a total of 78 protocol violations, and we have to count those people by what they were supposed to get, not what they did get."

"That's right," Mary shook her head. "I remember. That's the 'intention to treat' stuff, right?"

"Right."

"Katie, this is so great. I've got to call Tom and Dave and tell them!" She hurriedly gathered her things. "Thanks so much!"

"You're truly welcome."

Chapter 14

Reporting the Findings

Once all of the data have been collected and analyzed, the next step is to report the results of the study. The presentation of the results can take many forms, ranging from an informal report to colleagues to publication of the results in a peer-reviewed medical journal.

Typically, the first effort at reporting research results involves preparing an abstract (or summary) of the study that the researcher submits for consideration by a professional organization or scientific meeting. Once the abstract is accepted for presentation, the researcher will either prepare and present a brief oral presentation of the study findings or develop and display a poster that reports the study methodology and results. Once the research has been presented, the next step is to write a full manuscript for publication in the medical literature.

This chapter reviews each of these opportunities for presenting research results.

ABSTRACT PREPARATION AND SUBMISSION

Most major scientific research is initially reported by submitting an abstract to the meeting of a professional organization or to a state or national convention. This abstract is slightly different from the one found at the beginning of a published paper. The purpose of this abstract is to draw attention to the study so that the reviewers will select it for presentation. It specifically addresses only results that are directly related to the research question, and does so in a very condensed format. Because of space constraints (usually the abstract is restricted to around 250 to 300 words), the author limits the introduction, methodology, and conclusion sections. Instead, emphasis is placed on the presentation of results.

The specific format for this type of abstract is detailed in the call for abstracts put out by the sponsoring agency. The call for abstracts guidelines specify the word count, the font and size of the type, the specific headings that must be included, and the deadline date for submission. Calls for abstracts can be found in most major medical journals throughout the year.

How much information is contained in the abstract is related to the type of project that was done. For some research, the methods are equally as important as the results, so space must be carefully allocated to comply with the word limit. Most often an abstract will contain a one- or two-sentence introduction that clearly states the hypothesis or research question. This is followed by the methods section, which is limited to only key information about the type of research conducted. The results section is usually the longest portion of the abstract and often includes the total number of participants used in the analysis and a few of the important findings that support or refute the hypothesis. This is followed by the conclusion section, which is limited to only one or two sentences. Depending on the organization issuing the call for abstracts, tables or figures may or may not be allowed.

Once the abstract is submitted to the sponsoring agency, it is reviewed by a team of other authors and researchers, usually leaders in their respective fields, and graded in such areas as content and originality. Blinding reviewers to the identities of the authors helps ensure that the evaluation is unbiased, but not all organizations conduct blinded abstract reviews. The scores from the reviews are tallied and, based on those scores, certain abstracts are chosen for presentation at the group's state, national, or international convention. Once selected, the abstract can be placed into one of two categories: oral presentation or poster presentation.

ORAL PRESENTATIONS

The abstracts chosen for oral presentation are usually considered the best of the submissions. These authors are typically given 15 minutes to present the findings from their research projects. The format of the oral presentation usually follows the text of the abstract, but during the actual presentation it is possible to expand on specific sections and explain terms, equipment, and data a little more clearly.

The first 10 minutes of the presentation are designated for actual presentation of the scientific information. The remaining 5 minutes are set aside so that the audience can ask questions about the study or make constructive comments about the methodology or the conclusion. The opportunity to make an oral presentation of an abstract is a true honor for the researcher.

Because an oral presentation is made to a large audience, authors usually use slides for the presentation. Slide order, content, and format are left up to the authors, but it is expected that the presenter will cover the key components of the abstract, including the introduction, methods, results, and conclusions. Most presenters include other slides in the presentation, such as graphs, charts, or photos of the equipment or other tools used in the project.

While making an oral presentation of a study can be intimidating, it is also an excellent opportunity for the researcher to learn more about the project. The questions and comments generated by the audience are almost always helpful when it comes time to write the manuscript. Most of the people in the audience understand the research process, and offer their comments in a supportive manner.

POSTER PRESENTATION

Most national conventions limit the number of oral presentations because of time constraints. Since most meetings receive and accept more abstracts than can possibly be presented in oral form, many authors are given the opportunity to present their work in a poster format. A poster presentation is a static display of the components of the research project along with additional supporting documentation. Presenters are given a large bulletin board space in an exhibition hall or other specified area.

Most poster presentations include the various components of the abstract in an expanded format. The print used for the poster should be large, and photographs, graphs, charts, and sometimes even the actual equipment used in the study can also be displayed. Posters are meant to be self-explanatory, as the authors are not always at the posters during the times at which they are displayed.

Modern computer software has made poster development, layout, and production much easier. Most medical universities have departments that can produce posters. Posters can also be produced through local printing shops—which can be consulted for help in determining the poster format and layout. However, posters do not have to be high-tech. Some researchers simply print each section of their poster on plain white paper using a large font size.

MANUSCRIPT PREPARATION

Manuscript preparation is the last piece of the research puzzle. Many researchers find this to be the most challenging part of the research process, and because of that some research never gets beyond the development of an abstract for presentation. But, unless the researcher puts pen to paper and gets the study into print in a journal or magazine, no one outside of the researcher's organization and the few people who saw the abstract presentation will ever know about the project.

Putting a manuscript together begins with a decision on which journal or magazine would be most suitable for the project. There are a variety of publications to review. Some are more scientific, while others contain more general types of research studies. Once the researcher has decided on a journal, it is important to get a copy of that journal's author guidelines. These are usually published in the first issue of each year, and sometimes repeated several times throughout the year. For some journals it may be necessary to write directly to the publication or check the publisher's Internet Web site to get a copy of the instructions. The local medical library may also have information about various author guidelines. The Raymon H. Mulford library at the Medical College of Ohio maintains a Web site that provides instructions for authors from most medical journals (www.mco.edu/lib/instr/libinsta.html).

These guidelines or instructions contain information on how to format the manuscript, how many copies to submit, to whom to submit them, and the style and organization of the references within the manuscript. The guidelines also provide information about table formatting, page numbering, and author waivers that must be signed before the paper will be considered. Many journals also request that a computer diskette with a word processing version of the manuscript be submitted along with the paper copies. Submitting a manuscript without following the journal's guidelines will almost always result in an immediate rejection.

COMPONENTS OF A RESEARCH MANUSCRIPT

Whether the researcher is writing a manuscript for publication, a report for a company, or proposed changes for protocols or policies, it is important that certain key elements be included in the research manuscript to provide a foundation for the research findings. Any document discussing research findings should always include:

An abstract
An introduction
A methodology section
A results section
A discussion section
A conclusion

Depending on the type of manuscript being written, the length of each of these sections will vary, but the purpose will always remain the same.

The Introduction

The purpose of an introduction is to provide the reader with a brief synopsis of the importance of the project and to identify the research direction taken by the authors. The introduction should highlight the reason the project was necessary, using background information from the literature, and end with the hypothesis or research question. A review of the literature assembled during the project development phase will probably reveal some additional points to include in the introduction.

An introduction should always be brief—in most cases, no longer than one or two paragraphs. In all components of research writing it is important to be as concise as possible, always maintaining focus on the purpose of the section. The introduction, for example, is not the place to present findings, methodology, or implications of the project. Its purpose is to introduce some background information and the study hypothesis.

The researcher can learn more about introduction sections by reading other research articles and looking carefully at the introduction sections. Not all published articles are examples of good writing, but reviewing examples of both good and bad introductions will be helpful.

The Methodology Section

This is the section of the paper that contains detailed information about how the project was done. While it is not meant to provide step-by-step instructions, it should contain enough information about the data collection process and methods for analysis that a reader could repeat the study. Typically the level of detail in this section ranges from supplying information about any equipment that was used (including the manufacturer's name, the city and the state where the company is located, and model number if applicable) to listing the exact names of the statistical tests that were performed on the data.

The section usually begins with a description of the EMS service and/or hospital that participated in the project. Providing this information first establishes a foundation and allows readers to decide if the conclusions presented in the discussion section could be relevant to their service or area. Details about the service or hospital might include the number and types of EMS vehicles, the number of ALS and BLS providers, and the type of response system and any specialized dispatching protocols. This section might also report any hospital specialty services that respond upon EMS arrival (i.e., trauma team, chest pain team, etc.) or any elements unique to the EMS system, such as physician response to the scene.

Information about the patient selection criteria is usually included next in the methods section. If patients (including patient charts) were used in the study, then specific inclusion and exclusion criteria should be listed. The researcher should offer some explanation for any exclusion criteria that might seem unusual. For example, in a study on pediatric trauma it would be necessary to explain why an age limit of less than or equal to 15 years was used instead of 18 years. The explanation might be as simple as elimination of those trauma patients who were the drivers of motor vehicles. The methods section should also include information about the internal review board's approval of the study.

Next in the methodology section should be a discussion on the data collection process. When the study includes previously published or privately owned data collection forms or survey tools, it is important that proper credit be given in the manuscript. Examples of these types of data collection tools would include the Injury Severity Score,[12] TRISS methodology,[13] or any of a variety of learning inventories used in educational research. These acknowledgments can be made parenthetically or by using a reference number and providing the relevant information in the references at the end of the manuscript.

It might be helpful to list the information included on the data collection form, such as age, sex, type of injury, interventions, number of days in the hospital, or ultimate disposition. Or, if the data form is complicated, unique, or particularly short— or if the researcher just wants others to have access to it—the entire form can be submitted as a figure for inclusion in the manuscript.

The methods section usually concludes with a paragraph on the statistical tests that were used to analyze the data. This includes a discussion of the power calculation, the exact name of the statistical tests that were used, the alpha value used for determination of significance, and the computer software that was used to conduct the analysis.

As with the introduction section, the researcher can become better acquainted with methodology sections by reading other research articles. Again, these articles will likely provide examples of both good and bad writing and reporting styles.

The Results Section

The results section contains just what one would expect: the results. This section usually begins by identifying the total number of patients enrolled in the study or the number of charts that were reviewed. This provides the reader with a general idea of the magnitude of the project. Next the researcher reports the demographics of the subjects or participants. This is information such as the age, sex, and number of patients in each of the groups used for comparison, and other general descriptors about the study population. However, the investigator must be careful not to provide a level of demographic data that might make patients identifiable.

To reduce the wordiness that can occur when trying to report patient demographics, the researcher may consider presenting these data in a table. This reduces the volume of the text, and the researcher can direct the reader to the location of all of the data in one simple phrase: "See Table 1."

The bulk of the results section should focus on the data generated by the study, comparisons between study groups, and the results of the statistical tests that support or refute the null hypothesis. As with the demographics, when the data become too cumbersome to discuss in text form, the researcher should consider presenting them using tables or graphs. Most people find looking at tables or graphs more informative than reading words on a page, and tables and graphs can sometimes relate considerable information at just a glance. If graphs or tables are included, however, the reader still needs to be directed to their location and given information about their significance in the text.

The investigator should also report the statistical findings related to the data in the results section. Readers expect to see statistical findings, including P values and confidence intervals, when they read this section. Not including the statistical findings can reduce the credibility of the paper. The researcher must remember that failing to find statistical significance is, in some cases, just as important as finding statistical significance.

The researcher should also report unexpected or troublesome events in the results section. The investigator should be completely honest about the data, reporting such problems as patients who were lost from the study due to incomplete records, or instances of noncompliance with the study protocol that might affect the results. These data are part of the study results, and the reader must be informed of them and allowed to make decisions about how they might impact the study's findings.

When writing the results section of a paper, the researcher may want to consider developing an outline before actually putting pen to paper. An outline can assist in making sure all the pertinent findings are included as well in making sure the findings are all reported in some logical order. Developing the related graphs and tables before beginning to write the results section can also help the researcher to organize thoughts and reduce editing time.

The Discussion Section

The discussion is where the researcher explains what all the findings mean. This is the section where one draws inferences from the data, makes comparisons with other studies, and builds a case to support the findings. The investigator must be careful, however, to avoid editorializing.

First, the investigator should discuss the findings of the current study and how they might impact the patients, subjects, or system in which the study was done. The researcher should be sure to discuss all the pertinent data that were presented in the results section.

This discussion usually includes a review of the pertinent literature. The author should consider including literature that presents findings that are either similar or dissimilar to those of the current study, highlighting those articles that used similar methodology, and comparing and contrasting the results of those studies.

The discussion section should always include a paragraph or two on the limitations of the study. This is where the researcher tells the reader about the difficulties and shortcomings of the study. These can include anything from a patient population that was smaller than expected, to poor compliance with the research protocol, resulting in the loss of a high percentage of patients. The limitations section is important because it tells the reader that the researcher has critiqued his or her own work and identified potential weaknesses, and wants the reader to know what those weaknesses are. It also helps future researchers wanting to replicate the study by making them aware of these problems so that they can try to avoid them.

The Conclusion

The manuscript should end with a specific conclusion. Often this can be a restatement of the hypothesis or the null hypothesis, whichever was supported by the study. Or, if the data did not support a single, clear conclusion, this section might include two or three sentences indicating what the data at least suggest. When that is the case, the concluding statement might also call for more research into the subject.

Sometimes the conclusion is incorporated as the last paragraph of the discussion section; sometimes it is reported in its own section. This varies from journal to journal. The researcher will have to refer to the guidelines for authors to determine what each journal requires.

The Abstract

Even though the abstract is the first section of most written reports, it is usually the last section of the manuscript to be written. The purpose of this abstract is to provide the reader with a brief overview of the project, including the background, hypothesis or research question, methods, results, and conclusions. Writing this abstract is much easier than it sounds. Because the manuscript has already been written, the author may simply select key sentences from the various sections of the manuscript and assemble them into an abstract.

Most journals limit the number of words that can be used in the abstract. This means that the abstract is usually less than one page in length. In order to comply with the word limit, the author may forgo much of the background information and discussion section and focus mainly on the methods and the results. This allows readers to make some judgment about the importance of the study to their practices— or to their planned research projects—before reading the entire manuscript.

MANUSCRIPT SUBMISSION AND REVIEW

Once the manuscript is written, the review and publication process begins. Submission of a paper to a journal does not mean automatic acceptance. All truly scientific journals use the peer review process. In this process the manuscript is sent out to three or four experts on the research topic. These individuals evaluate the manuscript, make comments about the content, and ask questions about missing information or unclear statements. These individuals also recommend to the editor whether the paper should be accepted for publication. It is easy for the researcher to get discouraged during this review cycle. It can take several months to find out the fate of a manuscript.

Once the review process is completed, the researcher will receive a notice from the journal editor along with a copy of the reviewers' comments, including questions, suggestions, and reservations. Sometimes an editor will provide the author with the opportunity to revise the manuscript based on the reviewers' comments and resubmit the paper for publication. Other times the editor will send back the comments and a letter explaining that the manuscript is not suitable for the journal.

The researcher should always look over the reviewer comments. The researcher may not always agree with what was written, but the comments will be helpful in identifying areas where the manuscript can be made stronger. The comments will also help the researcher to avoid similar pitfalls when conducting his or her next study and writing the next manuscript.

Rejection from one medical journal does not mean that a research project was not successful, or that the paper is not suitable for publication. It simply means that one journal is not interested in publishing the paper. That may be because of the way the manuscript was written, because of methodological flaws in the study, or simply because the journal has been overwhelmed with similar studies. If a researcher receives a rejection letter from a medical journal, he or she should carefully consider the reviewers' comments, revise the paper as much as possible to address those concerns, and then identify another journal to which the paper can be submitted. Some papers are submitted to, reviewed by, and rejected by as many as three, four, or even more journals before ultimately being accepted for publication.

SUMMARY

Participating in the research process is very important, but equally important is reporting the findings so that others can benefit from the work. Research findings can be reported in informal reports, as abstracts submitted to and presented at professional meetings, and in manuscripts submitted for publication in peer-reviewed journals. To be successful in writing and publishing research, one must use the same tenacity and perseverance as was required for the research project itself. Research manuscripts follow a certain format, and the researcher should develop manuscripts following those standards and the guidelines published by specific medical journals. It is easy to get discouraged by the publication process, but the investigator must continue working toward the goal of publication. With hard work and practice, it will happen.

A Typical Experience
Part 12: Reporting the Findings

"Hello?" Tom usually didn't answer the phone when he was in bed, but whoever was calling was letting the phone ring on and on and on.

"Tom! They took it! They accepted the abstract!"

"Mary?" Tom tried to clear his head. He looked at the clock; it was just before noon. "Mary, I worked all night."

"I know, I'm sorry, but the mail just came. Our aspirin study was accepted for presentation at the state EMS conference!"

"Yee-haw," Tom said flatly. "Cool. Awesome. You're great. Good night."

"Don't you dare hang up on me!" Mary listened for a second. "Tom?" The line was dead. She hung up the phone. Then she picked it up again and dialed Timmy's number.

"So," he asked, "is it an oral presentation, or *just* a poster presentation?"

"Poster. But that's OK with me, I'm not sure I want to stand up in front of a crowd of people and present this. Not my first study, anyway."

"Mary," it seemed Timmy couldn't stand for her to have any joy, "it's only a state conference. It's no big deal. Our albuterol study was presented at the national emergency physicians' meeting."

Mary hung up the phone. No goodbye; no nothing. She wasn't going to let Tom and Timmy ruin this for her. She had worked hard to put the abstract together, and she was proud of what she had done. Trying to describe 18 months worth of work in 250 words wasn't an easy thing to do, and she didn't feel like they had helped that much, anyway. Timmy always had some kind of criticism, and Tom never said anything more than "that looks great to me." In truth, while Tom's approach made her feel better, Timmy's comments had probably been more useful. She decided to go down to the print shop that had produced the data forms and talk to someone about how to lay out and produce the poster.

"This is quite an impressive poster. Have you considered submitting it to one of the national meetings?"

Mary hadn't caught the man's name, but he was an emergency physician from somewhere. "No, I thought that was shooting too high for my first study."

"This is your first study ever?" The short, bald, but good-looking man was surprised. "This is very good. You really should consider submitting it to the ACEP or the NAEMSP meeting. There's also the Prehospital Care Research Forum group if you'd rather have a more EMS-ish audience. In any event, this deserves a larger audience."

"Thank you." Mary didn't know what else to say. "I'll certainly think about it."

"Do that, and don't wait too long to get a manuscript written. This is clearly publishable."

"Really? I hadn't thought much about that." Given the way things had been going with Tom and Timmy, Mary found the man's encouragement refreshing. "It's just a local study. Do you honestly think people would be interested?"

"It's a randomized, controlled, blinded clinical trial in EMS. Yes! People will be interested in it." The man gave Mary his business card, and told her to contact him if she needed help with anything.

Several other conference attendees who stopped by the poster offered positive comments. A few wondered aloud why it hadn't been accepted for oral presentation, and one other person had echoed the notion that Mary shouldn't delay in getting a manuscript submitted for publication.

That night, in her hotel room, she began outlining a paper on the hotel's stationary. Working through the introduction wasn't too hard because she still remembered most of what she'd found in the literature. When she got to the methods section, she decided it would be easier to work through that if she had all of her notes from those original planning meetings in front of her. Skipping to the results, she copied most of the information from her abstract, and then made a note to include tables. Under "discussion" she made a list:

    Aspirin common in EMS
        Based on ED/inpatient practices
        Not previously studied in field
    This study shows it works
        Mortality rate cut in half
        Treating 67 patients saves 1 additional life
    Limitations
        Only 1 system
        Only short-term survival measured
        Protocol violations

She looked over the list, and then added:

    Timmy

It took almost a month for Mary to finish the manuscript and then another 2 weeks for Tom and Dave to read over it and make suggestions. Finally, she had sent the required number of copies—all double-spaced, in 12-point type, on pages with wide margins—and a disk with a word processing version of the manuscript to the journal editor. The letter that acknowledged receipt of the package told her to expect the review to take 60 to 90 days. It had been 10 weeks. Mary opened the envelope, equally excited and scared. There was a cover letter with three or four attached sheets of paper. As she read through the letter, her expression didn't change.

"So?" Tom asked. They were getting along better now. They had been reassigned as partners and had been riding together for about 2 months.

Mary flipped through the remaining pages. "They want a bunch of changes made."

"But then they'll publish it?"

"I don't think that's a sure thing. The letter says they'll *reconsider* it." Mary stuffed the pages back in the envelope. "Maybe I should just send it somewhere else."

"Maybe, but it seems to me that they're telling you what they want. Is there something they asked for that you can't do?"

"Not really, but it'll be a lot of work." Mary pulled the pages back out of the envelope and passed them to Tom. "There's a bunch of other papers they want me to reference, but at the same time they say the discussion is too long. They also say there are some other limitations that I should address."

"OK, so it'll be some work, but at least you know exactly what they want you to do."

"I guess I just got my hopes up too high." Mary rubbed her eyes. "Maybe I need to think on it a while."

"You know," Tom knew how to close a deal, "this journal is way more prestigious than the one Timmy's study got published in."

Mary smiled. "OK, I've thought on it a while. I'll start the revisions tomorrow."

"Attagirl."

It was almost Thanksgiving, and Mary was looking forward to having a holiday with her family. It had been 8 months since her poster presentation, and more than a year since they had finished data collection. That meant it had been more than 2 years since they started data collection, and almost 3 years since she and Tom had that first conversation about him forgetting to give aspirin. She sometimes wondered if it was all worth it.

"Hey Timmy, have you seen this?" Mary was sitting at the Station I kitchen table when Timmy came in for his shift.

"What's that?" he asked as he walked over to look.

Mary slid the newest issue of an emergency medicine journal across the table. The second article listed on the cover was "Randomized controlled trial of prehospital aspirin for chest pain: Effect on mortality."

"Page 238," she said.

Timmy leafed through the pages. There it was. Mary's study that he had told her couldn't be done. Published.

"Congratulations." It was clearly an obligatory statement, void of any true emotion.

"Thanks, Timmy," Mary said, with a smug grin on her face. "Yep," she thought, "it *was* worth it." She folded her arms across her chest and tipped back in her chair. For a moment— actually, more than a moment—Timmy hoped she'd topple over backward.

Appendix 1

Frequently Asked Questions

HOW DO I PAY FOR THIS?

Finding the money to pay for research might be one of the hardest parts of the whole process. Established PhD researchers in medical schools and private laboratories spend a significant portion of their time trying to track down funding for their research projects. The good news is that most EMS research does not require millions—or even thousands—of dollars.

If a project is small enough, it may be possible to pay for it with "in-kind" contributions from the EMS system. In other words, the system won't have to put up any cash, but it will have to provide things like medical supplies, copier paper, and access to a copying machine. Another in-kind contribution that an EMS system can make is providing personnel by allowing EMS providers to work on a project while they are on duty. If a project is small enough, it may not require any actual cash.

If the project does require funding, there are several possible sources. If the study involves an evaluation of a medication, the company that produces that medication might be willing to provide funding. The same is true if the study is evaluating a specific piece of equipment. If a student or faculty member of a local university—or, better, medical school—can be recruited to help with the study, that institution might have some funding available. The EMS researcher can also request funding from charitable organizations, such as the local chapter of the Red Cross or Heart Association.

Finally, EMS researchers can pursue grant funding from both governmental and private agencies. Grant writing is an art in itself, but the researcher who develops this skill can seek funding from hundreds of agencies, ranging from charitable trusts to such governmental organizations as the Centers for Disease Control and the National Highway Traffic Safety Administration. Don't be discouraged by rejections from granting agencies. The competition is tough. Every experience—even the failures—helps the researcher to learn the process and to improve the grant request for the next time around.

IS MY QUESTION GOOD ENOUGH? IS IT REALLY IMPORTANT?

The simple answer is *yes!*

Certainly, some questions have more potential to profoundly change EMS than others, but all questions have value. If any one EMS person has a question, it is likely that somewhere around 27,328 other EMS people have the same question. It's just like being in school—there are no stupid questions.

It is guaranteed that someone will have reservations about any research question. Someone will doubt that it is important, someone will doubt that it makes any difference, someone will doubt that it's worth all the effort to get the answer. They're wrong!

It is important, though, to look carefully at the question and be sure that it is exactly the question the researcher intends to answer. It is also important to be sure that the question is specific, that it is a question that can be answered, and that the answer produced by the study will in fact be about the question that was asked. Remember, formulating the question, and then the hypothesis, is an integral part of the research process.

WHO CAN HELP ME WITH THE LITERATURE REVIEW?

Willie Sutton robbed banks because "that's where the money is." The library is where the literature is—and nobody knows more about libraries than librarians.

Even the most experienced researcher in the world can benefit from the help of a good librarian. Sure, the researcher can learn to do a literature search using computerized software, and can probably get copies of all of the articles if he or she has access to a local medical library. Yet, there are many "tricks" to getting a complete literature search, and the librarian knows those tricks better than anyone else does. Don't be afraid to ask for help; that's what librarians do. In fact, if a researcher goes into a library and tries to do the search by him- or herself, it is entirely likely that a librarian will come up and offer to help.

Other places to get help with the literature search include other researchers, particularly those associated with medical schools; other EMS providers; and the EMS medical director. While it's unlikely that any one person will be familiar with all of the literature about any given topic, someone might say, "Oh, I just read an article about that in. . . ." The researcher can then get that article and look at the references to see if they include other papers that might be of interest. Also, the medical director is likely to have access to at least one, if not all, of the popular emergency medicine journals, most of which publish an index of articles at the end of each year.

WHAT IF MY STUDY HAS ALREADY BEEN DONE?

While there isn't any reason to re-invent the wheel, there may be legitimate reasons for repeating a study that has already been done. Recall from Chapters 8 and 13 that all studies involve at least some degree of chance, which means there's at least some chance that the results of the study that has already been done are inaccurate. This is less likely if the study has been done 26 times using 19 different methodologies—but there aren't many things in EMS that have been studied 26 times.

There are other reasons to repeat studies, too. A study of ambulance response times in Washington, D.C., is probably not relevant to an EMS system in rural Alaska. A study of weather-related illness in the Upper Peninsula of Michigan is probably not relevant to an EMS system in New Mexico.

So the researcher has to look at the work that has been done and decide whether or not that work answers his or her question. If it does, and there are no circumstances that would make the researcher question the applicability of the results to his or her system, then it's probably not necessary to repeat the study. But if there are flaws in the methodology, or if there are only one or two studies about the topic, or if the studies that have been done cannot realistically be applied to the researcher's own system, then repeating the study is probably worthwhile.

ISN'T QA/QI THE SAME AS RESEARCH?

The simple answer is *no!*

Quality improvement data can be used to conduct research, but quality improvement activities are not, in and of themselves, research.

Research is designed to answer a specific question by testing a specific hypothesis. Most quality improvement programs do not set out to test a hypothesis. Instead, they collect data and then decide later what questions the data answer. Quality improvement asks, "What is our intubation success rate?" A research hypothesis would be, "Intubation success rates during night shifts are lower than success rates during day shifts." The QI data can be used to answer the question, but that's not why the QI program was initiated.

CAN'T I JUST DESCRIBE WHAT HAPPENS IN MY SYSTEM?

Yes, the researcher can choose to describe what happens in his or her EMS system. Descriptive research is one of the most basic types of research. Keep in mind, however, that descriptive research has inherent weaknesses. It does not test a hypothesis, and it can be affected by several different kinds of bias.

Descriptive research is worthwhile, and in fact a descriptive project might be exactly the right kind of project for the new researcher embarking on his or her first research experience. If any given EMS system does something unique—has a special staffing configuration, or deals with a type of response that is uncommon in other areas—it is certainly worthwhile to share those experiences and the things that have been learned from them with others. For example, describing the response to the World Trade Center or Oklahoma City bombings would be good descriptive research projects that could be helpful to other systems. It would be impossible to have a randomized, controlled trial of responses to bombings, so descriptive research may be the only way to get at such information.

Eventually, though, the EMS researcher should graduate from descriptive studies into studies that actually test hypotheses. There's a definite limit to the number of worthwhile descriptive studies that can come out of any one EMS system—but there is no limit to the number of hypotheses that can be tested.

WHO CAN HELP ME DESIGN THE STUDY?

An experienced researcher can provide the best help with designing a study, but there are several other resources, too.

An experienced researcher can give the new researcher some insights into the types of problems that might be encountered, the unforeseen difficulties common in research projects, and potential solutions for addressing—or maybe even heading off—those problems. It doesn't have to be a researcher who has published dozens of papers, just someone who has been through the process two or three times and has an understanding of how things go.

Other EMS providers can help, too. Even if they are unfamiliar with the research process, they are familiar with EMS, particularly in their systems. They can help refine the hypothesis, and they can help determine the best way to collect the data. They can also warn the researcher about potential problems. Don't discount the reservations that other EMS providers might have. Even if they're not that enthusiastic about research, their concerns will be real and the EMS researcher can avoid a lot of headaches by addressing those concerns early in the research process.

Another source of help in designing a study is the existing literature. The researcher will have already read all of the studies that have been published about the topic of interest, but there might be other studies that can help in designing the methodology. A well-designed study comparing subcutaneous epinephrine to IV epinephrine for anaphylaxis might serve as a useful model when designing a study comparing sublingual nitroglycerin to nitroglycerin paste.

WE DON'T HAVE AN IRB. WHERE DO I GET APPROVAL?

This is actually a big issue for EMS researchers. The best solution is to ask a local hospital or university IRB to review and approve the research proposal. Some institutions will provide this service for any researcher in the area; some will only review proposals from researchers affiliated with a certain institution; some will do it for free, others will charge a fee. If the EMS researcher can recruit a member of the hospital staff or university faculty as a co-investigator, the likelihood of having access to that facility's IRB is improved.

An EMS system can set up its own IRB, but this is a much more difficult task than it might seem. The National Institutes of Health has specific guidelines for IRBs that must be followed.

It is important to note that IRBs are not intended to obstruct research. They play a valuable role in the research process: They ensure that all research activities are ethical. Most researchers would not knowingly embark on an unethical project. The problem is that most researchers are very passionate about their interests, and it is difficult for them to objectively evaluate their own work. The IRB helps the researcher to be sure that the study is ethical.

IS IT REALLY POSSIBLE TO GET INFORMED CONSENT?

Yes. It can be difficult, it can take time, and it can be burdensome, but it *is* possible. Some of the studies referenced earlier in this book involved obtaining informed consent. There are several ways to accomplish this, including the two-step process described by Zehner et al. in their study of terbutaline and albuterol.[5]

Much like the role of the IRB, the role of informed consent is to help protect patients. Patients have a right to know when they are being experimented on. Even if the researcher truly believes that the experimental intervention is "better" for the patient, it is still experimental. The patient has a right to know, and a right to choose not to participate.

The IRB can be particularly helpful in developing the method of obtaining informed consent.

HOW DO I GET OTHERS TO HELP ME COLLECT DATA?

Say "please" and "thank you." Really. Often the EMS researcher designs a study, plans the implementation, and then calls a meeting to *tell* the field providers what they are expected to do and what data they are expected to collect. The best way to get colleagues to help with a project is to involve them early on, listen to their comments and concerns, and ask them to help with the project. If the study is one that most of the other EMS providers believe answers a worthwhile question and will help them provide better care or service to patients, most of them will be willing to help.

Bribery works too. Some researchers have a philosophical objection to bribing people to get their help. Philosophically, all EMS providers should be willing to help with research as a part of advancing the profession. In fact, if you asked most EMS providers outright, they'd agree with that. But philosophy has little to do with how anyone acts at 3:20 in the morning when they're cold and tired and taking care of another respiratory distress patient. A "free" day off for the person who enrolls the most patients, on the other hand, will be pretty enticing right about then.

When all the data have been collected, say "thank you." Don't just say it to the one person who won the free day off, say it to everyone. Even say it to the people who didn't enroll anyone. Saying "thank you" may or may not get you more help in the future. Not saying "thank you" will guarantee that fewer people will help you next time around.

WHERE CAN I GET HELP WITH DATA ANALYSIS?

Chapters 8 and 13 contain more complete information about data analysis and where to find help. Most importantly, the researcher should not try to do the analysis him- or herself, unless he or she also just happens to be a trained statistician or epidemiologist.

If the researcher has access to a medical school, or any other university, there will probably be statisticians employed there who can help with the analysis. Most people in academic settings need to participate in research in order to get promoted, so they have a real interest in helping with such things. However, the researcher should always contact the statistician or epidemiologist early in the design of the study. That person will be much more likely to agree to help at that stage. The researcher should not expect anyone to be happy if he or she shows up with a box of already collected data and says, "Hey, can you analyze this for me?"

Community colleges with strong math departments, local governments, and even some businesses (insurance companies, for example) may have people on staff who can help with statistical analysis. These people, too, will want to be contacted early in the process.

TO WHOM SHOULD I REPORT MY RESULTS?

Everyone!

First, if the study addressed an issue that is important to a specific EMS system, the results should be reported to the people in that system—both the administrators and the field providers. The reporting of the results could include a formal presentation at a meeting of the staff, or a simple written report distributed in memo form.

Next, report the results to all of the other people who helped to get the study done. This may include the medical director, people from the community or other EMS systems, anyone or any agency that provided funding, and so on. These people need to know what the study found, and sharing the results is particularly important if the researcher will ever need their help for a future project.

Finally, the researcher should present the results to the larger EMS and/or emergency medicine community. This is done by preparing an abstract for submission to a state, regional, or national meeting, and by preparing a complete manuscript for publication in an EMS or emergency medicine journal. Chapter 14 contains more information on this topic.

WHAT IF I FIND THE EXACT OPPOSITE OF WHAT I EXPECT?

Take a long, critical look at the hypothesis, at the methodology, at the data, and at the results. Do they all make sense? If so, the researcher simply must accept that the world is not exactly as he or she thought. That's OK. Finding the opposite of what was expected is not failure. The question has been answered, and that's the point of doing research. It is still important to present the results to all of the appropriate parties.

HOW LONG WILL ALL THIS TAKE?

The amount of time necessary to complete a research project varies considerably depending on the project. Some projects can be conceived, planned, implemented, and completed over the course of a weekend. Others take years to complete. In general, stronger, more important, more complicated studies take more time.

One mistake many researchers make is not considering the amount of time necessary to plan and design a study, or the time necessary to analyze the data and prepare a manuscript. Instead, they focus only on the time required to actually collect the data. Sometimes data collection represents only a very small portion of the time necessary to complete a study—particularly in retrospective studies where the data already exist.

If time commitment is an issue, the researcher should try to estimate the amount of time necessary to complete each of the steps discussed earlier in this book. Usually, the entire process will take more time than what the researcher estimates. After careful evaluation, one might estimate that a study will require 1 month to plan and develop, 3 months for data collection, 1 month for analysis, and 1 month to write an abstract and prepare a manuscript. In reality, it will probably take 9 to 12 months to complete that project, not 6 months.

The researcher should not be intimidated by the time requirements. A 9-month project is usually not 9 months of 8-hour days. Instead, it is 2 hours today, 4 hours next Thursday, and so on. Depending on how much time the researcher can dedicate to a study, it may be possible to complete relatively complex studies in a few weeks to a few months. Conversely, it may take a year to complete a relatively simple project if the researcher only spends 1 or 2 hours a week working on it.

IS IT REALLY WORTH ALL THE EFFORT?

Absolutely. Even a project that turns out to be a complete failure—one that completely falls apart and never gets finished—is an opportunity to learn about the science of EMS. There is still very little science to what we do. Every little bit of learning helps.

The EMS provider who undertakes a research project *may* advance his or her career, achieve some measure of status among his or her colleagues, gain rapport with physicians, get to travel to meetings in exotic places, or achieve fame through publication. Without doubt, though, the EMS provider who undertakes a research project *will* become a better EMS provider. And that's what it's really all about—improving the prehospital care of patients.

Appendix 2

Glossary

Abstract: A brief summary of a study, usually structured to identify the hypothesis, the methodology, the results, and the conclusions.

Allocation: The method by which study subjects are assigned to an intervention.

Alpha value (α):   The amount of chance of type I error that a study will accept. An alpha value of 0.05 represents a 5 percent chance of type I error.

Analysis of variance (ANOVA):   A statistical test that compares means among three or more groups.

Anecdotal: Learned through nonscientific personal experience.

Assent: A parent's agreement to his or her child's participation in a study.

Basic science: Laboratory research; sometimes called *bench research.*

Beneficence: A principle of research ethics that states the research must result in some good for society.

Beta (β):   The amount of chance of type II error a study is willing to accept; sometimes called *power.* A beta of 0.8 represents an error rate of 20 percent, or a power of 80 percent.

Bias: Something that systematically affects a study's results, whether intentional or unintentional.

Blinded review: A process in which the reviewers of abstracts or manuscripts do not know who the author is or where the study was conducted.

Blinded study: A study in which the subjects do not know whether they are assigned to the intervention or control group.

Call for abstracts: An announcement of a scientific meeting inviting investigators to submit summaries of their work.

Case control study: A study that identifies subjects with and without a particular outcome, and then looks back to see the rate of exposure to the study factor in the two groups.

Case report: A journal article that discusses individual clinical experiences.

Categorical data: Descriptive data or qualitative data

Chi-square (χ^2) test: A test that examines associations between groups described using categorical data. The chi-square test does not test cause-and-effect relationships.

Clinically significant: A research finding that would be meaningful to patients.

Clinical research: Research exploring a patient care intervention.

Cohort study: A study that compares outcomes in two or more groups that have different exposures to the study factor.

Comparative study: A study that examines outcomes in more than one group of subjects.

Confidence interval: A range in which the true mean or proportion probably exists. A 95 percent confidence interval of 1 to 4 would mean that, in 95 out of 100 studies, the finding would be somewhere between 1 and 4.

Confounding variable: Something that might affect a study's outcome that is not part of the study factor. Age could be a confounding variable in a study comparing the heights of male and female children.

Consent: A subject's agreement to participate in a study.

Contingency table: Usually a two-by-two table showing the association between groups of categorical data.

Continuous data: Data that are measured numerically.

Control group: A study group that is not exposed to the study factor.

Controlled study: A study in which one or more groups are not exposed to the study factor.

Cross-sectional study: A study that examines the state of things at a particular moment in time, or among a particular group of subjects.

Data point: An item of information that is collected during a study.

Data safety monitoring board: An independent group that intermittently reviews a study's data to ensure that the study is not causing harm.

Demographics: The characteristics of study subjects, such as age or sex.

Dependent variable: The outcome variable; the thing that the study factor may affect.

Descriptive study: A study that does not test a hypothesis.

Discussion: The section of a research manuscript that describes what the results mean.

Double-blind: A study in which the investigators and the subjects do not know whether they are assigned to the intervention or control group.

Educational research: Research that explores differing approaches to training EMS providers.

Effect size: The amount of difference a researcher expects to see between the intervention and the control groups.

Error: Incorrect findings or conclusions.

Ethical: Adhering to the principles of respect, beneficence, and justice.

Exclusion criteria: Specific reasons for not including subjects in a study.

Exempt: A study that does not require full review by an IRB. Typically, the IRB chair must decide whether a study is exempt; the researcher should not make that determination.

Expedited review: A process by which the IRB can quickly review a study protocol, usually involving fewer reviewers and requiring less time than full IRB review.

Experimental protocol: A meticulous, step-by-step description of the study process, including the subject inclusion and exclusion criteria, allocation technique, randomization scheme, and data collection process.

Experimental research: Research that tests a hypothesis.

Figure: A drawing, photograph, chart, or graph included in a manuscript to provide a visual representation of data.

FINER: An acronym describing the qualities of a good research question: feasible, interesting, novel, ethical, and relevant.

Fisher's exact test: A test of association for categorical data when the contingency table contains small numbers.

Frequency: The number of times an observation or finding occurs.

Frequency table: A table reporting the number of times several different observations or findings occur.

Guidelines for authors: Instructions on how to prepare an abstract or manuscript, usually distributed with a call for abstracts, or by journals to prospective authors.

Hawthorne effect: The observation that people behave differently when they know they are being watched.

Helsinki Declaration of 1964:   A document codifying many ethical principles, including those regarding research on human subjects.

Historical prospective study: A before-and-after study.

Hypothesis: A statement of fact that a study attempts to prove or disprove.

Inclusion criteria: Specific reasons for including subjects in a study.

Independent variable: The study factor; the thing(s) that might affect the dependent or outcome variable.

Informed consent: Agreement to participate in a study after being informed of the potential risks, benefits, and alternatives.

Instructions for authors: See Guidelines for authors.

Internal review board (IRB):   Also called the institutional review board or ethics panel; a group of people who review a study before it is implemented to ensure that it is ethical.

Interval data: Continuous data that do not have an absolute zero.

Intervention: The study factor.

Investigator: A person who conducts research.

Journal: A periodical that publishes research findings.

Justice: A principle of ethics that requires all study participants to bear the potential risks and benefits equally.

Kappa (κ): A statistical test that measures agreement.

Key words or phrases: Words or phrases used to index manuscripts and abstracts to facilitate their identification during literature searches.

Kruskal-Wallis test: A test that compares median rankings among three or more groups.

Laboratory experiment: A study conducted in a controlled environment.

Limitations: Shortcomings of a study, or things that might affect the usefulness of the results.

Literature: The collection of scientific publications about a topic.

Literature search: The process of identifying relevant scientific publications about a topic.

Manuscript: A paper describing a study, from beginning to end, that is submitted to a journal for publication.

Mean: The average.

Median: The middle value in a set of data.

Medical subject heading (MeSH heading): An identifier used to index published papers to facilitate their identification during a literature search. Also called MeSH term.

Methodology: The step-by-step process by which a study is conducted. See Experimental protocol.

Minimal risk: A condition in which the risks associated with a study are no more than the risks a subject might encounter in day-to-day life.

Multicenter trial: A study conducted at more than one location. Multicenter trials can enroll larger numbers of subjects and minimize the effects of things that might be unique to one specific location.

Nominal data: Categorical data that have no relative value (e.g., horse; cow; lamb; hog).

Null hypothesis: A statement that is the opposite of the hypothesis. True experiments test the null hypothesis.

Nuremberg Code of 1947: A document codifying many ethical principles, including those regarding research on human subjects.

Observational research: Nonexperimental research.

Oral presentation: A didactic presentation of study results, usual lasting only 10 to 15 minutes.

Ordinal data: Categorical data that have relative value (e.g., tiny, small, normal, big, huge).

Outcome variable: The dependent variable; the thing the independent variable or study factor might affect.

Paired t-test: A statistical test examining the mean difference between two groups.

Peer review: A process by which the researcher's colleagues and/or contemporaries review and comment on a study.

PICO: An acronym describing a well-written research question—patients, intervention, comparison group; outcome.

Pilot study: A small preliminary study intended to test the experimental protocol before full-fledged implementation of a study.

Placebo: An inactive drug or intervention.

Poster presentation: A static display reporting the results of a research project.

Power calculation: A prestudy attempt to determine the number of subjects needed for a study.

Predictor variable: A study factor, usually used in conjunction with a retrospective study.

Principal investigator: The primary or lead researcher on a project.

Prospective: A study that starts now and collects data from now until some point in the future.

Proxy: A person empowered to make decisions on someone else's behalf.

P value: A result reported by a statistical test that indicates the likelihood that the study results occurred by chance alone. A P value of 0.03 means that the results would occur by chance alone in only 3 out of every 100 identical studies.

Qualitative data: Data that are not measured numerically; categorical data.

Quantitative data: Data that are measured numerically; continuous data.

Quasi-experimental research: A comparative study in which the study factor is not randomized.

Random: Without order, happening completely by chance.

Randomized controlled trial: A comparative study in which allocation to the intervention or control group is completely random.

Range: A measurement of the spread of a data set; the difference between the lowest and the highest value.

Ratio data: Continuous data that could have an absolute zero.

Repeated measures: Special statistical techniques used when several measurements of the same data point are collected from the same subject.

Research question: The question that the study attempts to answer.

Respect for persons: A principle of ethics that requires subjects be treated as self-sufficient, self-directed individuals.

Results: The findings of a study.

Retrospective: A study that examines existing data that were collected at some point in the past.

Review article: A nonresearch paper that summarizes all of the existing literature on a topic.

Sample size: The number of subjects needed for a study to be able to achieve statistical significance.

Scientific meeting: A gathering of professionals at which the findings of original research are presented.

Search strategy: The key words and MeSH headings used to identify the literature related to a topic.

Setting: The environment in which the study is conducted.

Standard deviation: A measure of the spread of a data set; conceptually, the average difference between any single data point and the mean value of all data points.

Statistically significant: Findings that are unlikely to have occurred by chance alone.

Statistical test: Any of a number of mathematical calculations designed to determine the likelihood of differences between sets of data occurring by chance alone.

Statistician: A person skilled at selecting and applying statistical tests.

Study factor: The independent variable; the thing that the investigator believes might affect the outcome variable.

Study population: The group of subjects eligible for inclusion in a study.

Study subject: Individual enrolled in a study.

Survey: A written questionnaire distributed to study participants.

Systems research: Research exploring different approaches to providing emergency medical services.

Trade magazine: A periodical that publishes articles and news items, not peer-reviewed scientific research.

***t*-test:**   A statistical test that compares the means of two groups.

Type I error: Also called alpha error; finding a statistically significant difference between groups even though the difference occurred simply by chance.

Type II error: Also called beta error; failing to find a statistically significant difference between groups even though the difference did not occur simply by chance.

Variable: Something that the researcher thinks might affect the outcome of a study, or might itself be affected by the trial; one of the data points the researcher records.

Waiver of consent: A process by which the IRB can allow subjects to be recruited for a study without having to give written informed consent; studies involving unresponsive patients may qualify for waiver of consent.

Wilcoxon rank sign test: A statistical test examining changes in median rankings.

Wilcoxon rank sum test: A statistical test comparing the median rankings of two groups.

Appendix 3

Mentor Organizations and Scientific Meetings

PREHOSPITAL CARE RESEARCH FORUM

The mission of the PCRF is "the promotion, education, and dissemination of prehospital research." The PCRF is not a membership organization, but instead a working coalition of EMS professionals.

Each year, the PCRF publishes an international call for abstracts. Abstracts are received from providers, clinicians, educators, and administrators from around the world. Abstracts in the categories of clinical, systems, management, and personnel are presented at the Annual EMS Today Conference; abstracts in the category of education are presented at the National Association of EMS Educators Symposium. The PCRF also offers a research workshop, often in conjunction with these and other meetings.

More information about the PCRF can be found at www.pcrf.mednet.ucla.edu.

NATIONAL ASSOCIATION OF EMS PHYSICIANS

The mission of NAEMSP is to be "an organization of physicians and other professionals who provide leadership and foster excellence in out-of-hospital emergency medical services." NAEMSP has a standing research committee.

At the annual meeting of NAEMSP, attendees have the opportunity to network, introduce new ideas and policies, and present scientific papers. Both oral and poster research presentations are accepted. NAEMSP also offers a research workshop at its annual meeting.

More information about NAEMSP can be found at www.naemsp.org.

SOCIETY FOR ACADEMIC EMERGENCY MEDICINE

The mission of SAEM is "to improve patient care by advancing research and education in emergency medicine."

The SAEM annual meeting is held each May. Over 500 research studies are selected for presentation each year. They are presented in oral and poster format, and include studies relating to emergency medical services. SAEM also sponsors regional meetings in various locations across the United States.

More information about SAEM can be found at www.saem.org.

AMERICAN COLLEGE OF EMERGENCY PHYSICIANS

The mission of ACEP is "to support quality emergency medical care and to promote the interests of emergency physicians." ACEP has both an EMS section and an emergency medicine research section.

The annual ACEP Research Forum provides an important opportunity to present and discuss original research at a national gathering of researchers and teachers of emergency medicine. Both oral and poster presentations are invited. There is usually a large volume of EMS-related research.

More information about ACEP can be found at www.acep.org.

Appendix 4
EMS-Related Journals

SPECIFIC TO OUT-OF-HOSPITAL CARE

Air Medical Journal

The official journal of the Air & Surface Transport Nurses Association, the Air Medical Physician Association, the Association of Air Medical Services, the National EMS Pilots Association, and the National Flight Paramedics Association.

Editors: David Dries, MD, and Renee S. Holleran, RN, PhD
11830 Westline Industrial Drive
St. Louis, MO 63146-3318
Tel: (800) 453-4351
Fax: (314) 432-1158
E-mail: journal.service@mosby.com

Prehospital and Disaster Medicine

The official journal of the World Association for Disaster and Emergency Medicine.

Editor: Marvin L. Birnbaum, MD, PhD
E5/613 Clinical Sciences Center
600 Highland Avenue
Madison, WI 53792-6733 USA
Tel and fax: (608) 263-9641
E-mail: mlb@medicine.wisc.edu
Web site: www.wadem.org

Prehospital Emergency Care

The official journal of the National Association of EMS Physicians, The National Association of State EMS Directors, and the National Association of EMS Educators.

Editor: James J. Menegazzi, PhD
230 McKee Place
Pittsburgh, PA 15213
Tel: (412) 578-3235
Fax: (412) 681-5319
E-mail: menegazz+@pitt.edu
Web site: www.naemsp.org

GENERAL EMERGENCY MEDICINE

Academic Emergency Medicine

The official journal of the Society for Academic Emergency Medicine.

Editorial Office
901 North Washington Avenue
Lansing, MI 48906
Tel: (517) 485-5484
Fax: (517) 485-0801
Web site: www.saem.org

American Journal of Emergency Medicine

Editorial Office
The American Journal of Emergency Medicine
3800 Reservoir Road NW
Washington, DC 20007
Web site: www.wbsaunders.com

Annals of Emergency Medicine

The official journal of the American College of Emergency Physicians.

Editorial Office
PO Box 619911
Dallas, TX 75261-9911
Tel: (800) 803-1403
Fax: (972) 580-0051
Web site: www.acep.org

Emergency Medicine Journal

Editorial Office
BMA House
Tavistock Square
London WC1H 9JR
Tel: +44 (0)20 7383 6795
Fax: +44 (0)20 7383 6668
Web site: www.bmjpg.com

European Journal of Emergency Medicine

The official journal of the European Society for Emergency Medicine.

Editorial Office
Department of Emergency Medicine
Universitaire Ziekenhuizen Leuven
UZ Gasthuisberg, Herestraat 49
3000 Leuven, Belgium
Tel: (+32) 16 34 3927
Fax: (+32) 16 34 3894
Web site: www.euro-emergencymed.com

Journal of Emergency Medicine

The official journal of the American Academy of Emergency Medicine and the Canadian Association of Emergency Physicians.

Editorial Office
University of California, San Diego, Medical Center, 8676
200 West Arbor Drive
San Diego, CA 92103-8676
Web site: www.aaem.org

Appendix 5
LITERATURE SEARCH SOFTWARE

There are many searchable databases containing indexes to the medical literature. In the United States, the National Library of Medicine maintains Medline®, which is perhaps the most commonly searched database. In fact, the phrase *medline search* is sometimes used generically to mean *literature search*. In the UK, EMBASE is the more popular database. Other searchable databases include:

AgeLine
AIDSLINE
AIDSDRUGS
AIDSTRIALS
BIOETHICSLINE
CancerLIT
CINAHL
HealthDigest
HealthSTAR
PsycINFO

Each of these databases includes specific types of reference material, which may or may not be of interest to the EMS researcher depending on the study topic and research question.

There are also many search engines available for exploring these databases. Not all search engines are linked to all of the databases, so the researcher must choose the search engine carefully.

FREE SEARCH ENGINES AVAILABLE ON THE INTERNET

- *PubMed*—www.ncbi.nlm.nih.gov/PubMed
- *Grateful Med*—igm.nlm.nih.gov (uses PubMed engine)
- *HealthGate*—www.healthgate.com (limited free access)
- *DIMDI* (German)—www.nacsis.ac.jp (limited free access, can switch to English-language version)

FEE-BASED/SUBSCRIPTION SEARCH ENGINES

- *OVID*—www.ovid.com
- *STN*—www.stn.com
- *BIDS* (UK)—www.bids.com
- *NACSIS* (Japanese)—www.nacsis.ac.jp
- *DataStar/DIALOG*—www.dialog.com

There are likely other databases and search engines of which we are not aware. The researcher should be able to identify those resources through an Internet search, or by contacting a local medical library.

Appendix 6

Statistical Analysis Software

STATISTIX

Analytical Software
PO Box 12185
Tallahassee, FL 32317
Tel: (800) 933-7879
Fax: (850) 894-1134
Web site: www.statistix.com

SAS

Worldwide Corporate Headquarters
SAS Institute Inc.
SAS Campus Drive
Cary, NC 27513-2414
Tel: (919) 677-8000
Fax: (919) 677-4444
Web site: www.sas.com

SPSS

Corporate Headquarters
SPSS Inc.
233 S. Wacker Drive, 11th Floor
Chicago, IL 60606-6307
Tel: (312) 651-3000
Fax: (312) 651-3668
Web site: www.spss.com

EPI-INFO

Centers for Disease Control
Atlanta, GA
Tel: (770) 488-8440
Fax: (770) 488-8456
Web site: www.cdc.gov/epiinfo

STATVIEW

SAS Institute Inc.
Attn: StatView Sales and Marketing
SAS Campus Drive
Cary, NC 27513
Tel: (919) 677-8000
Fax: (919) 677-4444
Web site: www.statview.com

Appendix 7

CITED LITERATURE AND SUGGESTED READING

CITED LITERATURE

1. Grossman E, Messerli FH, Grodziki T, Kowey P. Should a moratorium be placed on sublingual nifedipine capsules given for hypertensive emergencies and pseudoemergencies? *JAMA*. 1996;276:1328–1331.
2. Sakles JC, Laurin EG, Rantapaa AA, Panacek EA. Airway management in the emergency department: a one-year study of 610 tracheal intubations. *Ann Emerg Med*. 1998;31:325–332.
3. Chan D, Goldberg RM, Mason J, Chan L. Backboard versus mattress splint immobilization: a comparison of symptoms generated. *J Emerg Med*. 1996; 14:293–298.
4. Mattox KL, Bickell W, Pepe PE, et al. Prospective MAST study in 911 patients. *J Trauma*. 1989;29:1104–1112.
5. Zehner WJ, Scott JM, Iannolo PM, et al. Terbutaline vs albuterol for out-of-hospital respiratory distress: randomized, double-blind trial. *Acad Emerg Med*. 1995;2:686–691.
6. Totten VY, Sugarman DB. Respiratory effects of spinal immobilization. *Prehosp Emerg Care*. 1999;3:347–352.
7. Lo B, Feigal D, Cummins S, Hulley SB. Addressing Ethical Issues. In: Hulley SB, Cumming SR, eds. *Designing Clinical Research*. Baltimore, MD: Williams & Wilkins; 1988:151–157.
8. US Dept of Health and Human Services Rules and Regulations. *Title 45: Code of Federal Regulations: Part 46;* Revised as of March 8, 1983. Washington, DC: US Department of Health and Human Services; 1983.
9. Levine RJ. *Ethics and Regulation of Clinical Research*. Baltimore, MD: Urban & Schwarzenberg; 1986.
10. National Commission for the Protection of Human Subjects of Biomedical and Behavioral Research. *The Belmont Report: Ethical Principles and Guidelines for the Protection of Human Subjects of Research:* DHEW Publication No. (OS) 78-0012. Washington, DC: US Government Printing Office; 1978.
11. Human Subjects Committee. *Manual of Procedures:* Richard C. Powell, PhD Chairman. Tucson, AZ: University of Arizona; 1995.

12. Baker S, O'Neill B, Haddon W, Long W. The injury severity score: a method for describing patients with multiple injuries and evaluating emergency care. *J Trauma*. 1974;14:187–196.
13. Boyd C, Tolson M, Copes W. Evaluating trauma care: the TRISS method. *J Trauma*. 1987;27:370–378.

SUGGESTED READING

Babbs CF, Tacker MM. Writing a scientific paper prior to the research. *Am J Emerg Med.* 1985;3:360–363.
Byrne DW. *Publishing Your Medical Research Paper*. Baltimore, MD: Williams & Wilkins; 1998.
Cuddy PG, Elenbaas RM, Elenbaas JK. Evaluating the medical literature: part I: abstract, introduction, methods. *Ann Emerg Med*. 1983;12:549–555.
Elenbaas JK, Cuddy PG, Elenbaas RM. Evaluating the medical literature: part III: results and discussion. *Ann Emerg Med*. 1983;12:679–686.
Elenbaas RM, Elenbaas JK, Cuddy PG. Evaluating the medical literature: part II: statistical analysis. *Ann Emerg Med*. 1983;12:610–620.
Gonick L, Smith W. *The Cartoon Guide to Statistics*. New York, NY: HarperCollins; 1993.
Hulley SB, Cumming SR (eds). *Designing Clinical Research*. Baltimore, MD: Williams & Wilkins; 1988.
Mandel J. *The Statistical Analysis of Experimental Data*. New York, NY: Dover; 1963.
Sackett DL, Haynes RB, Guyatt GH, Tugwell P. *Clinical Epidemiology: A Basic Science for Clinical Medicine*. 2nd ed. Boston, MA: Little, Brown; 1991.
Weldon KL. *Statistics, A Conceptual Approach*. Englewood Cliffs, NJ: Prentice-Hall; 1986.

INDEX